Presented To:

_____

From:

_____

Date:

_____

More Than A Conqueror

A Step-by-Step Guide

to

Showing Cancer Who's Boss!

LITA P. WARD

CANNONPUBLISHING

More Than A Conqueror

A Step-by-Step Guide

to

Showing Cancer Who's Boss!

LITA P. WARD

CANNONPUBLISHING

Copyright © 2017 by Lita P. Ward

Cannon Publishing
P.O. Box 1298
Greenville, NC 27835
Office: 888-502-2228
www.cannonpublishing.net

Printed in the United States of America

First Printing, 2017
ISBN – 13: 978-0692897331
ISBN – 10: 069289733X

Ordering Information: Books may be purchased in quantity and/or special sales by contacting Lita P. Ward at www.litaward.org or 252-944-6708.

DEDICATION

To every person who has courageously fought this
fight and those who have cared for someone
in the fight.

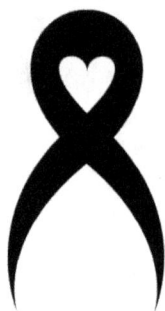

LESLEY'S TRIBUTE

In honor of my last radiation treatment on
June 13, 2014, my sister, Lesley Rodgers posted
the following on social media:

*"I don't like the term 'survivor.' I prefer
'conqueror.' To me, survivor seems like
something blew in and out like a storm, and
somehow you made it through; I feel like this
thing came by surprise and you defeated it!!!*

*On today as you ring that bell, I want you to not
only feel like a Survivor....I want you to feel like a
Conqueror!*

*Through this experience, I have learned what I
needed to learn; to appreciate every little thing,
to see the world from a different perspective. You
have shown me what it is to be a Conqueror; to
not let anything or anyone get me down. Just to
put it in God's hands and He will take care of it.*

*I am so proud of you! I love you and I am so
happy you conquered this!"*

ACKNOWLEDGMENTS

I want to thank God for healing my body, and allowing me more time with family, friends and the opportunity to complete my Kingdom assignments.

Thank you to my husband, Victor J. Ward, for being my caregiver and greatest supporter, who prayed for me and loved me back to health.

To my children, Cecelia, Antonio, Derell, Rakita and Jamika, thank you for your love and prayers. To my grandchildren, thank you for motivating me to become well so I could see each of you grow up. To my many God sons and daughters, thank you for your prayers.

Special thanks to my sisters and brother, Lesley, DeLynn, Linda, Nikki and Roderick; my mothers, Annette Purvis, Glendora Lee and Jeanette Sheppard; Dr. Mahvish Muzaffar, Dr. Lacy Hobgood, my doctors and nurses at Leo Jenkins Cancer Center, Vidant Medical Center and Eastern Radiologists Breast Imaging Center; my pastor, Bishop Claudie H. Wilkins and wife, Missionary Deloris Wilkins, and Little Thankful Praise & Presence Ministry Church family; my staff and coworkers at the University of Mount Olive; and all of my family and friends.

To my Carla, but known to many as Carla R. Cannon, The Trailblazer...Thank you for your innate ability and ministry for being a midwife.

Your push and vision for this project has helped me deliver not just a book, but a message of hope and healing!

Special Recognition to Inspiring Warriors...
Apostle Vonner Hogan, Evangelist Veronica Morgan, Brenda Jenkins, Lizzie Everett, Louise Rodgers, Valerie Williams, Pamela Freeman, Nedra Harris, Belva Wallace, Sonia Pruitt, Dora Faison, Muriel Hines Jones, Anna Barnhill, Marilyn Perkins and Juanita Williams Wiggins.

In Special Memory...
Clara Purvis, my beloved grandmother
Nancy Barnhill
Myra Cooper
Cassandra "Val" Lloyd Ward

TABLE OF CONTENTS

FOREWORD

Prognosis: (*noun*) a forecast of the likely course of a disease or ailment

Many years ago, a patient told me that he wanted to know what his condition was going to be; that even if I couldn't cure the disease, I should be able to tell him what was going to happen to him next. Since that time, I have come to appreciate the value of giving my patients a prognosis. It is never enough to simply give a diagnosis, although making the correct diagnosis is critical to the process of healing. In order to solve a problem, one must first define the problem. A good physician can tell you what the problem is – diagnosis; while a great physician can tell you, what is going to happen next – prognosis.

Lita P. Ward's book does an excellent job of telling patients and their families what is going to happen next, and does so in language that is easy to follow and understand. Her chapters are laid out in a logical sequence from receiving a cancer diagnosis to facing treatment decisions to managing side effects of those treatments. Throughout, she never loses sight of the patient – the person facing the diagnosis – and offers encouragement, support, advice, and most important of all, hope.

My hope for you is that you are able to use this book as reference material to guide you or your loved one through your cancer treatment.

Lacy Hobgood MD, FACP, FAAP

Greenville, NC

A CONQUEROR'S GUIDE TO GETTING THE MOST OUT OF THIS BOOK

When I was diagnosed with Stage IIA breast cancer, I was given a lot of information consisting of pamphlets, brochures, magazines, books and websites. It was overwhelming and there were times I did not feel up to researching and digging for answers, tips and suggestions regarding cancer, chemotherapy, radiation and relative topics.

During this time, a dear friend of mine, on several occasions, insisted that I write a book and share my story regarding breast cancer. Her advice was that I not only share my story, but also provide pertinent information to help someone else who may have just heard the dreadful words, "You have cancer."

After much encouragement and consideration, I decided to move forward in my research, not knowing the information I found would not only benefit me, but many others as well. I admit I am not a medical professional; therefore, I have relied on the information and sources provided to me from my firsthand experiences, as well as the medical team assigned to me during my process. The information within these pages are not intended to diagnose, treat, or cure any medical condition, or dispense medical advice.

Now here's how to get the most out of this book. At the end of each chapter, there will be Conqueror's Notes created for you to write essential information, such as questions to ask your doctor at your visits, names of doctors, or your thoughts and feelings. These spaces are designed especially for you to journal. Also, at the end of the book I have incorporated pages to notate your personal journey. I encourage you to utilize these pages, because who knows, one day, you may take on the task of writing your own book or sharing your story in some way. And the content within your journaling could be a great starting point! Not only will these entries be healing for you, but also for someone else. Isn't that what life should be about? Your greatest test is when you can bless or help someone else while you are going through your own storm.

As you utilize the guide, I advise that you do not skip ahead without journaling. This tool is an invaluable way of walking you through your journey to recovery. At the end of the guide, you will find Appendices to use for referencing and support.

Finally, my prayer and intent for the Conqueror's Guidebook is to help:

A. Those who have been recently diagnosed;

B. Those who have overcome any medical condition;

C. And family, friends and loved ones of those who may currently be in the fight of their life.

This guide will provide them with hope, a sense of peace and the assurance that they can and will do more than just survive cancer; but thrive to be a Conqueror and show cancer who is boss!

Who Will Benefit the Most From This Guide?

A. Those with a current diagnosis: This guide provides insight on what one can expect from the different methods of treatments, medications, to side effects and how to cope with the various phases of the diagnosis.

B. Those who have overcome any medical condition: For you, this guide will offer encouragement to keep fighting and take charge of your health. It will inspire and remind you of the Conqueror's spirit within you.

C. Family, friends and loved ones of those who may currently be in the fight of their life. Naturally, it is hard to watch someone you love go through any hardship, especially sickness. This guide will also offer insight on what your loved one will experience as well as answer any questions you may have as you walk through this process with them.

1

YOU HAVE CANCER

*N*ever in a million years did I believe that I would ever hear these words, "I am sorry to have to tell you this, but you have cancer." But on September 9, 2013, which was my 18th wedding anniversary, I did hear them and it shook me to my core. Months before, I was getting in physical shape by attending a boot camp through Elite Fitness, owned and operated by Crystal White. I was eating better and working diligently to improve my lifestyle since I would be turning the big 5-0 in another six months or so. But at one boot camp session in late July on a hot, late afternoon, I noticed that I just could not keep up with the group. Even though some of my workout partners were half my age, usually I was at least able to finish the training course. Oh, and her courses were ruthless, consisting of lunges, burpees, sprints and lifting! But on that day, I became extremely fatigued rather quickly and decided to go home early that day. I didn't think any more of it, chalking it up to my body's reaction to an antibiotic given to me by my doctor for a minor ailment. Besides, it was hot and humid, so I decided to call it a day and go home. I would finish strong that next week. But next week never came. I just didn't feel good and decided to sit out that camp and wait for the next one.

One month later in August of 2013, my husband and I had just gone to bed and settled down for the night. Lately, I was always tired and exercise had become non-existent. When I turned over in bed to get comfortable and lay on my favorite right side of my body, my nightgown caught me rather tightly under my left arm and neck, so I reached under my left armpit to pull it down. But when I did, I felt a lump under my armpit and it startled me because it was rather large in size. Immediately, I asked my husband to feel what I was feeling and we both agreed that I would go to the doctor to get it checked out. I called the next day to make an appointment with my primary care physician, Dr. Lacy Hobgood, but he wasn't available, so I saw another doctor in the same facility. We went through the routine of questioning of whether I had hit it on something or bumped into anything. I thought the questioning was absurd because the knot was so far under my arm. How could I have it on something and cause and injury? I just wanted her to tell me right then that it was nothing and it would go away. But instead, the doctor said she would give me a referral to have a mammogram done. I must be honest here; in my heart, I knew what it was. I just didn't know how bad or serious it was. I became very angry with myself because I did not do self-examinations on a regular basis. I believe that if I had, I would have discovered the lump sooner.

I remember attending church the Sunday before the mammography appointment and having one of my church sisters, Tara Counts, who happens to be an RN, check it for me. We went into the ladies' restroom and I showed her where to feel. I knew that she could not tell me one way or another of what it was, but just having the support of a friend was what I needed and wanted at the time. She said the same as the doctor that I should have it examined, but to trust God and she would be praying for me. I asked the church to pray for me and my mind kept going back to what if it was cancer or what could I have done differently since my last mammogram.

Well, on September 3rd, less than a week before our 18th wedding anniversary, I had a mammogram and an ultrasound core biopsy done at Eastern Radiologists Breast Imaging Center. Even though this health scare was happening, we were still planning to spend a few days in Myrtle Beach, South Carolina. I love the beach, the waves and the water, so I was looking forward to getting away, spending much needed private time with my husband and feeling the sand between my toes. Monday rolled around and even though the test results were in the back of my mind, I was in a decent mood, putting the finishing touches on our packing. Since we would be gone for a few days, I decided to go by my mother's house and make sure she had everything she would need while we were away. My cell phone rang that afternoon as I was leaving her house, and it was Eastern Radiologists' office. The nurse on the phone wanted me to come in and discuss my results with the doctor, not make an appointment, but come in that same day. I took a deep breath and told her that I could get there around 3:00PM. Before I could call my husband to tell him about my appointment, Dr. Hobgood, my primary care physician called, asking if Eastern Radiologists had contacted me to come into their office. I responded, "Yes and I have an appointment at 3:00PM." I knew then without a doubt that it was not going to be good news. I braced myself and called my husband Victor and told him that I needed him to go with me to the doctor to get these test results. Of course, he reassured me that everything was all right, but I knew that it wasn't, as far as these test results were concerned.

When we arrived at the doctor's office, waiting to be called back was sheer torture. But when my name was called, I hoped it was a mistake and they meant to call someone else's name. I just wasn't ready to hear what the doctor had to say.

Slowly, I got out of my seat and we followed the nurse. The nurse took us into this nicely furnished room with soft lighting, comfortable seating and a coffee table with magazines and Kleenex tissues and told us that the doctor would be right in. I know it's weird that I mention the tissues, but the sight of them made me think this is the room where they tell patients they have cancer. Why else would there be Kleenex tissues here? I thought about all the other women who had sat on this same chair hearing what I was about to here. I prayed to God that He would just allow me to survive and be able to tell my story.

There was a knock at the door and in walked the doctor and her assistant, Dr. Ericka Griffin, a beautiful and petite African American young woman, with a warm smile and bright pretty eyes. She could sense that I was terrified and anxious, so she got right down to business. Once she greeted us, she told me that the mass was a malignant tumor and cancerous. I found out later that the medical terminology was Stage IIA invasive ductal carcinoma; triple negative breast cancer.

When I actually heard the word "cancer", initially, I refused to believe it. Denial had set in. But this was my eighteenth wedding anniversary and I exercised and ate right! I had my entire life ahead of me with grandchildren to enjoy! All of these thoughts of why and how began to bombard my mind. I did not have time to deal with this type of sickness. I had too much to do!

Almost choking on my words, I stammered, "What do you mean I have cancer?" The doctor's words numbed all my senses. It was like I wasn't there and she was not talking to me. She could not have been talking to me. All I could feel was my husband's hand caressing my back, trying to reassure me that everything would be okay. Again, I just could not believe this was happening to me. I kept the tears and emotions at bay and asked her, "Now what? What is my next step and will I be alright?" I no longer wanted to hear about the cancer; just how to get rid of it and out of my body. No matter how spiritual I was, at the end of the day, I was not ready to die. I wanted to live. I still had too much purpose and vision left inside of me.

She assured me that if I followed the regimen of chemotherapy, surgery and radiation given to me by the team of doctors at Leo Jenkins Cancer Center, I would be healthy again and able to look back at this moment and see where the Lord had brought me from. Even her assistant said that they would be praying for me. Once given instructions on my next appointment with Leo Jenkins Cancer Center, we thanked Dr. Griffin and her assistant for their kind words and prayers and left the building.

Dazed by the dreaded news, my husband and I walked to the car. I felt like I had been kicked in my stomach. How was I supposed to tell my children that I had cancer? How was I going to tell my mom, my sisters, my coworkers? How was I supposed to work? There was no way I could be out of work for an extended period of time. We had bills to pay and I enjoyed going to work.

Many questions and concerns raced through my mind as we drove home. Then the floodgates opened and my tears rushed from my eyes. I couldn't hold it back any longer. I was terrified of the big "C"! For many, it had become a death sentence, one of suffering, pain and demise. I was afraid that God would not heal me; I was afraid that I had not caught it soon enough and literally when I had surgery, I would be told that it was too late and it was only a matter of time before I would die.

When we arrived at the house, my husband walked me into our bedroom and he told me that we were going to pray. As we stood in the middle of our bedroom, he took both of my hands into his and he began to pray for our family and me. I have heard my husband pray before because he prayed all the time. But as he prayed for me, it wasn't like all the other prayers I had heard him pray. He prayed so fervently that his voice began to sound like my pastor's voice and instead of opening my

13

eyes, secretly I peeked to see who was standing in front of me. When he was finished praying, I had the confidence that everything was going to be all right. I knew that there would be good days and some not so good, but we would get through them together.

We finished packing for our trip and left that next day for Myrtle Beach, South Carolina. We refused to allow this news to dampen our spirits and we had the greatest getaway ever. I enjoyed every moment of our trip, because I didn't know when we would be able to visit again. We walked on the beach with our toes in the sand, well I did. My husband was skeptical about his toes touching anything. We visited as many places as we could; ate my favorite foods like seafood and even visited the amusement park. To my amazement and Victor's, I got on this crazy ride called the Sling Shot, which shot us up in the air, about 300 feet. The view was absolutely beautiful, seeing the lights and stars as far as the human eye could see. Purposely, I had fun and refused to worry about the days to come, as well as their challenges. But I did know that we would be back to enjoy ourselves and when we did, I would be cancer-free, ready to celebrate life.

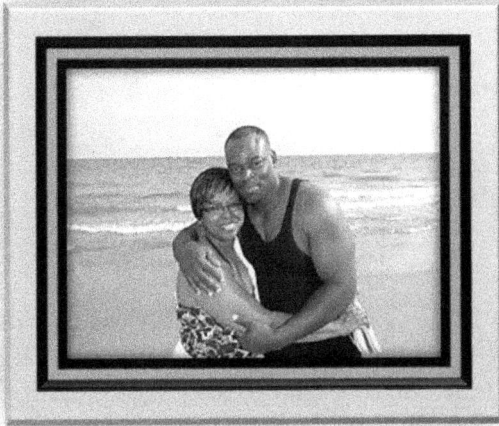

Myrtle Beach, SC
The Day After Receiving My Diagnosis
September 10, 2013

We were unsure of the tasks ahead, but we were confident in our love for one another and God's love for us. We made the decision to enjoy ourselves for the time we had. Enjoy every moment; life has a way of pushing you to not sweat the small stuff. There are a lot of days I wish I could do over, but we know that's impossible. So, instead of regretting and wishing, make the next moment, day, minute and hour count. Live life to the fullest; you only get one.

A Word of Encouragement

Currently Diagnosed – *Though it may if feel as if you are in the fight of your life, you can and will recover. This is not a death sentence; so, don't give up, but fight to live and live to fight!*

Conqueror – *I know you vividly remember when you received your diagnosis and the emotions you felt. So, I encourage you to share your story, use your God-given gifts and help someone else who may be experiencing what you have made it through.*

Caregiver – *If your loved one has just received a diagnosis, I am sure you feel a sense of helplessness. Please know you do not have to find the right words to say or do anything; just be there and offer your support and love.*

Conqueror's Notes

"Don't panic. I'm with you. There's no need to fear for I'm your God. I'll give you strength. I'll help you. I'll hold you steady; keep a firm grip on you." Isaiah 41:10 (MSG)

_____

_____

_____

_____

_____

_____

_____

_____

_____

_____

_____

_____

Conqueror's Notes

"Don't panic. I'm with you. There's no need to fear for I'm your God. I'll give you strength. I'll help you. I'll hold you steady; keep a firm grip on you." Isaiah 41:10 (MSG)

_____

_____

_____

_____

_____

_____

_____

_____

_____

_____

_____

_____

Conqueror's Notes

"Don't panic. I'm with you. There's no need to fear for I'm your God. I'll give you strength. I'll help you. I'll hold you steady; keep a firm grip on you." Isaiah 41:10 (MSG)

_____

_____

_____

_____

_____

_____

_____

_____

_____

_____

_____

2

YOUR BELIEF SYSTEM

When entering into a battle, one must prepare their mind, body and spirit, if you want to win the war. I am a firm believer that life and death is in the power of our tongues; therefore, to beat cancer or any disease, it is pertinent to speak healing regardless of doctor reports, tests, or actual feelings. Even now, after being cancer-free since June 2015, I still must speak healing over my body because of the risk or chance of reoccurrence.

It is extremely important to have a good attitude and outlook on life and your prognosis. Once you receive the diagnosis, then you should be working on having a positive prognosis. I made up in my mind that I would not walk around looking sick or hopeless. If I was going to be bald, then I was going to be the prettiest and baddest bald headed woman you ever laid eyes on. I refused to allow cancer to make me feel unattractive. I believed that I was pretty whether I had hair or not; hair never defined me, so why allow the lack thereof now to do it?

I remember standing in front of my bathroom mirror, shaving my head, watching my hair fill the sink, as tears filled my eyes. As my vision became blurred, so did my thoughts. Emotions of sorrow, loss and embarrassment swirled in my mind. But I kept saying to myself, "You can get through this. The hair will grow back." As I tried to convince myself, my husband walked into the bathroom and saw what I was doing. Immediately, I thought about covering my head. But before I could even react, he gently took the razor out of my hand and began to gently shave my head for me. It became a beautiful moment of compassion and intimacy between us. At that very moment, I was grateful again to have him in my corner. Soon thereafter, I posted a picture of my newly shaven head on Facebook. My status under that picture was "I am not brave or courageous; I am just a believer." I believed that if God allowed this to happen to me, He would also take care of me. That is what I believed and still do. This chapter is not just about Christianity, but it is also about being positive, positive in your thinking and speaking. Having a good and positive attitude is half the battle. You have every right to complain, but what good would it do? It won't help make the cancer go away or help you feel better. But it will get in your spirit, and cause things to be harder to bear. Most importantly, it will do nothing positive,

22

but more than likely make you miserable and depressed.

You may not consider yourself a spiritual person, but you really are. We are comprised of three parts, mind, body and spirit. The Bible tells us in 1 Thessalonians 5:23 that we were all created with three basic parts: a spirit, a soul, and a body:

"And the very God of peace sanctify you wholly; and I pray God your whole spirit and soul and body be preserved blameless unto the coming of our Lord Jesus Christ."
1 Thessalonians 5:23 (KJV)

But our deepest and most hidden part of our being is our spirit. And by our spirit we can contact the spiritual realm. No other creature was created with this third part, the spirit. By our spirit, God is real to us and we can contact Him, receive Him, and fellowship with Him. I advise you to tap into your spirituality. I believe it was and is prayer that brought my healing and is keeping me cancer-free. I had so many people praying for me and not just from my local church and fellowship, but from everywhere. When you are sick or troubled, you do not care who is praying as long as someone is praying and that God hears those prayers.

I prayed for myself and kept the Holy Scriptures and positive affirmations before me all the time.

23

On one of my work computer monitor's is the statement… "Faith sees, the invisible, believes the incredible, and receives the impossible." I received this from one of my coworkers, Jennifer Merritt one day through an email and it has remained on my monitor since then. I was given an acronym of the word **H.O.P.E.** from my pastor, Bishop Claudie H. Wilkins, which meant "**H**ave **O**nly **P**ositive **E**xpectations. I kept that taped to my mirror at home to read aloud daily. I quoted Scriptures of healing and hope; one in particular has become my testimony:

> ***"It is good for me that I have been afflicted; that I might learn thy statutes."***
> **Psalm 119:71 (KJV)**

I must admit that having cancer increased my prayer life and caused me to pursue the knowledge of God's Word and to trust and obey the Word of God. I even realized that this sickness was never about me, but it was about God. Why and how could I say this? Because I believe that it was allowed to come and to teach me things about God that I could not have learned any other way. God used this to teach me His Word and to build my faith so that I would end up closer to Him than I was before the cancer. And guess what? It did just that! Also, now I can share my testimony and story of what I went through, how I was able to endure and live. I can give hope from a personal account, not one of what I heard or read about. I can tell and show others that cancer does not have to be a death sentence.

I see God, my heavenly Father as a pair of bookends. He said that He is the Alpha and the Omega, the Beginning and the Ending. And He is the Author and Finisher of my faith. Therefore, He was with me and kept me from start to finish, from the beginning and the ending of cancer or any trial I may have experienced or will experience. Everything that I may encounter and experience was and is in between those book ends, so if I start out with Him in the beginning of it and finish with Him in the ending of it, what a powerful story of the stuff in between I will have to share with others! So why worry about the middle of it when you already know the ending will be in your favor and for your benefit?

I was talking to someone from the Greenville's Chapter of the American Cancer Society and I told her that once I began to be grateful for being selected as a candidate for a miracle, my attitude changed. I then started to thank God for allowing me to know Him as a Healer and Restorer. I complained less and expected to be healed. This did not happen overnight, but it was a process. Even cancer was a part of my process with the end result of growth in my faith and spiritual maturity. Everything we encounter is part of our process to be better and do better in this life.

To get you started in thinking and speaking positive, here are some positive affirmations:

1. I may have cancer, but it does not have me or define me.

2. Miracles happen every day; therefore, I am expecting my miracle of healing.

3. I will beat this and it will not beat me!

4. I am healthy and healed. I give thanks for my full recovery.

5. I am not just a survivor, but I am more than a conqueror because my inner strength comes from above.

According to what you may be seeing or feeling at this moment, these affirmations may not be true or evident, but just keep saying them. That is what faith is really all about, speaking things that are not true as if they are true. But please trust and believe, one day, they will be true! For the Bible says in Hebrews 11:1, "Now faith is the substance of things hoped for, the evidence of things not seen" and in Romans 10:17 "so then faith cometh by hearing, and hearing by the word of God."

When I speak these affirmations, and hear the words of healing, life and possibility, I am repelling fear and speaking faith into my situation. I hear these words and I begin to believe what I am speaking and hearing. If I hear it enough and believe it enough, surely it will begin to manifest in my body. Here again is the importance of understanding that we are made of three parts, mind, body and spirit. What I say to my mind will eventually get into my spirit and then my body will react! This goes for positive and negative thoughts and speech; therefore, speak life to yourself and believe it will come to pass.

Feel free to use the affirmations I have shared, but also take the time to write your own. When you write your affirmations, write them in present tense. Write as though you are experiencing what you desire *right now*. Moreover, make them short and to the point. Following this method will help you to recall them and make it easier to remember and recall. Now start affirming your positives!

1. I am _____

2. I am _____

3. I am _____

4. I will _____

5. I can_____

There is no specific amount of affirmations you should have, but what I do know is that they work. Whatever your care plan or regimen may consist of, you will need strength for the journey. Affirmations and prayer have proven that this is the first place to start, ensuring peace of mind and inner strength that will surprise you and those around you. In the Appendices section, I have provided 10 Affirmations for fear, depression and anxiety, accompanied with Scripture references.

Many days I didn't feel strong, but words and thoughts of healing and peace helped me through the day and night. Sometimes your toughest moments will occur at night, when the world is asleep and your meds have you up with insomnia. Instead of allowing negative thoughts and feelings to overtake your peace of mind, pull out your affirmations and read them or grab a Bible, which is full of hope, love, peace and strength. Those of us, who read the Bible on a regular basis knows that if you have problems falling asleep, grab a Bible and watch what happens next. Seriously!

Remember that your tongue has the power of life and death (Proverbs 18:21). Isn't it empowering to know that you have been freely given and graced to possess authority and dominion over sickness and death merely by the words you speak and choose to believe?

I could have easily allowed negativity to take over my thoughts, but what good or benefit would that have caused? It is just as easy to be and think positive than it is to do the opposite. Besides, thinking negatively affects your entire body. The common term is labeled as "stress" which we unknowingly bring upon ourselves often.

Finally, the Scripture Isaiah 53:5 was embroidered on a pink blanket and presented to me by my UMO staff (picture below). Please understand that scripture is not a magic formula or just positive words to recite or reflect on. The Holy Scriptures are the living words of God and even more so, they are Jesus Christ, the Living Word (John 1:1, 14). I believe that with all my being that His words are spirit and life.

"But he was wounded for our transgressions, he was bruised for our iniquities: the chastisement of our peace was upon him; and with his stripes we are healed."
Isaiah 53:5 (KJV)

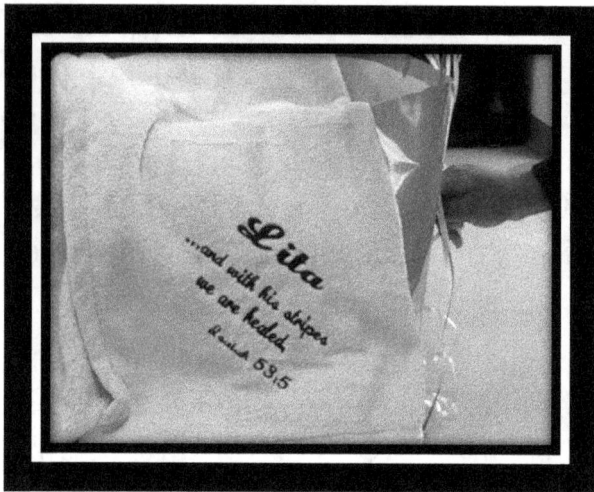

Gift from University of Mount Olive at Washington Staff in October, 2013

When you have the mentality that I may have cancer, but cancer does not have me, then you declare it until it becomes true and manifests itself right before your eyes. And today, here I stand, healed, grateful and excited about the future.

A Word of Encouragement

Currently Diagnosed – *Your words have power; therefore, speak life and positive things to yourself on a regular basis. Don't allow self-pity and fear to overtake you! You can get through this!*

Conqueror – *By now, you know how important it is to have and keep a positive mindset. I hope you continue to utilize your affirmations and believe that whatever comes your way will be handled; because you are more than a conqueror!*

Caregiver – *At this point, it is extremely important for you to speak life and hope to your loved one. If you do not know exactly what to say, just make sure you don't speak negative things. Your loved one does not need to be reminded of how Cousin Jimmy or Aunt Sue passed away from cancer, or how your coworker only made it past one month after chemotherapy. Help them fight and let them know that you will be right there to help them fight!*

Conqueror's Notes

"I know what I'm doing. I have it all planned out - plans to take care of you, not abandon you, plans to give you the future you hope for." Jeremiah 29:11 (MSG)

_____

_____

_____

_____

_____

_____

_____

_____

_____

_____

_____

_____

_____

_____

_____

Conqueror's Notes

"I know what I'm doing. I have it all planned out - plans to take care of you, not abandon you, plans to give you the future you hope for." Jeremiah 29:11 (MSG)

_____

_____

_____

_____

_____

_____

_____

_____

_____

_____

_____

_____

_____

_____

_____

Conqueror's Notes

"I know what I'm doing. I have it all planned out - plans to take care of you, not abandon you, plans to give you the future you hope for." Jeremiah 29:11 (MSG)

_____

_____

_____

_____

_____

_____

_____

_____

_____

_____

_____

_____

_____

_____

3

SHARING YOUR NEWS

I wasn't up for telling too many people at once. I knew my immediate family; children, mothers and sisters would need to know as soon as possible. Why? They could and would be my greatest support during the entire ordeal. I remember calling my sister DeLynn and sharing it with her over the phone. I knew that I could count her to be strong and tell Mama Glen and my other sisters. I assured her that I would be all right; besides I was the Big Sister and I had to be okay. I could tell that she was crying over the phone, but she held it together and let me know that whatever I needed they would be there for me and they were. There were days that my house needed cleaning and they were right there, Lesley leading the way. Baby sister Nikki (Tenika) is the cook of the family, so she would make me special dishes when asked. She even did a t-shirt fundraiser for me called *Sisters Supporting Sisters*. When they couldn't physically be there, I knew they were praying for me and would do whatever I asked. Even times when I was in the hospital, I didn't want them to come and see me in pain. You may think that was selfish of me, and yes, I must agree. But you must do what works best for you. I remember seeing a picture of myself while in the hospital and I could not believe that I was that sick. I hope that when you look back over your experience, you will be amazed and grateful to see how well you have progressed.

When it comes to family and friends wanting to do things for you, allow them. Not only does it help you cope, but also it helps them just as much. It can be just as hard on them as it is on you. No one wants to see his or her family member suffering; therefore, when they can do something physically, whether it is cooking, cleaning, conducting a fundraiser or just there to hold your hand, be grateful that you have someone there who cares.

But when it came to telling my children who were grown, I did not have the heart to, so my husband did it for me. He was able to do it without being emotional, explaining to them the doctor's report and reminding them that I was a fighter. Sharing the news with my mom wasn't hard because I knew she would be one of my greatest cheerleaders and supporters. I knew that I would be able to tell her when I was afraid, worried, or in pain. She would just look at me and say, "Little Girl, you are going to be all right. You are strong and God answers prayer."

Because I worked, I knew that I would need to share the news with my coworkers, my supervisor and human resources. I consider my coworkers friends, but instead of telling my entire staff, I broke the news to two of my most trusted coworkers first, Donna Waters and Stacy House. I remember returning to work from our Myrtle Beach vacation, and I asked to meet with both of them in my office. They came in, sat down across from me and I told them that I had something to tell them. I explained that I had been to the doctor, received a mammogram and that I had cancer. I really tried to be strong and not cry, but that did not work out too well. But one of the remarkable things about friends is that they will cry along with you. I expressed my fears and told them that I would need their help on those days I may be too sick to work due to chemotherapy treatments. Of course, they reassured me that they would do whatever I needed. My entire staff at the time, including Travis Kinsey and Robyn Schwartz, was so wonderful and supportive throughout the entire year of my recovery. Robyn made me homemade chicken noodle soup and placed it in several containers, which I could freeze and eat whenever I had the taste for it. In October of that year, my staff gave me a party with a beautiful cupcake cake shaped into the breast cancer awareness pink ribbon along with a blanket embroidered with my name and healing scripture of Isaiah 53:5.

My supervisor, Dean Lisa Nuesell and University of Mount Olive Human Resources department, Cordelia Wilcox and Russell Hopkins were extremely supportive as well; allowing me to work from home, get to my appointments, and sending constant prayers and gifts of cards, blankets, etc. I could go on and on about my University of Mount Olive family, consisting of fellow directors, staff, faculty, adjuncts and students who gave me invaluable support and encouragement during my fight with cancer and during recovery.

It is extremely important to have colleagues who are genuinely concerned about your wellbeing. One day I was talking with our Human Resources Director Cordelia Wilcox and she asked me if I had enrolled in our Allstate Benefits' Critical Illness insurance. I had completely forgotten that I had bought this insurance at least a year before my diagnosis. I contacted the insurance company and after providing them with proof of diagnosis, the company sent me a check in a lump sum. It was a blessing and I would recommend this type of insurance to anyone. One never knows when they too may be stricken with a critical illness and these types of benefits can assist you with bills and ongoing medications.

When it was time to share with my church family, the timing was sort of ironic. For the past couple of months, our women's ministry, the DOVES had been organizing a breast cancer awareness program. We thought it would be great to raise money and donate it to the local Relay for Life chapter since several of our members had been stricken with breast cancer in the past and currently. It was on a Saturday afternoon in October and some of the ladies and I were putting up pink ribbon signs, pink tissue paper streamers, and decorations for the service. I remember feeling overwhelmed and overcome by emotions, because I knew that I had cancer and would be facing so much in the days, months and year to come. The only people aware of this were my immediate family and pastor, Bishop Wilkins and his wife, Lady Deloris. My sister DeLynn kept asking me if I was okay and I put on a brave face and kept it moving. Before the service started, I nonchalantly told my friend, Angela Adams that I had been diagnosed with breast cancer. Stunned by my words, her face displayed disbelief and I could see tears forming in her eyes, but again, I put on my brave face and kept it moving. It shocked her and I even felt bad for telling her in the manner that I did, but in reality, it may not come out the way you plan. After I said it, I wished I had kept it to myself and told her later. But because of the anxiety I was experiencing, I just let the cat out of the bag, per se.

I had invited several breast cancer conquerors to be on the program and it turned out well. It was very inspiring and encouraging to hear the conquerors' experiences and how they had made it back to their healthy selves. Close to the end, when it was time for my remarks, I thought it would be a great idea to tell the congregation about my diagnosis. In this manner, I would be able to tell everyone at one time and it would be out in the open. There were people there who knew and understood what I was about to encounter so they encouraged me, gave me tips and I was glad my news was finally out.

Whenever you decide to share your diagnosis, remember that it is your prerogative as to who you share it with and how much information is shared. I was fortunate to have an amazing support system. Even my students were supportive when I explained to them that I would not be teaching for an extended period of time. Their well-wishes, thoughts and prayers helped me through many dark days and nights. But if you find yourself not able to tell someone, then allow your family or someone close to you to do it for you. In this journey, you will need support from others. Do not be afraid to ask for it; you will be extremely glad you did and so will your family and friends.

Another method of sharing and getting moral support for me was through social media. Through Facebook on October 28, 2013, I created a private group entitled "Lita's Journey to Wholeness (Isaiah 53:5)" where I enlisted about 50 people who I knew would pray and encourage not just me, but also my family in the rough times. In this private space, I could post updates, emotions, and whatever was laid on my heart and mind at the time to write. Many of group members always posted encouraging words, pictures, tips, suggestions or remedies for some of the side effects I experienced. Two members would post almost every day, Lakita Corey of Georgia and Tenita Johnson of Michigan; what a blessing! These two were amazing as well as all the others who helped me on this journey. Another friend of mine and member of my group, Christina Takahashi who now lives in Pennsylvania sent me an email back in March 2014, which completely touched my heart and spirit. When I told her about the cancer in September, she began growing her hair to contribute it to her local "Locks of Love" organization in honor of me and my journey. There are some things God does and allows which totally humbles you; this was at the top of my list.

This mode of communication became my method for venting and sharing through blogging or journaling about the experience. I had no idea that I would utilize it later as a resource for a book! It has also become a way for me to look back and see just how blessed I am to have been able to conqueror cancer and have all those wonderful family members and friends to supporting me.

A Word of Encouragement

Currently Diagnosed – *It is okay to take your time on when to share your diagnosis and to whom to share it with.*

Conqueror – *If you haven't thought about sharing your story, why not? And if you blogged or did journaling during your process, then you are off to a great start. If not, it is never too late to start.*

Caregiver – *Before you share your loved one's diagnosis with anyone, please get their permission. They may not be ready to receive the attention or care from others and want to be private at this point. Talk to them first.*

Conqueror's Notes

"Have I not commanded you? Be strong and courageous. Do not be terrified; do not be discouraged, for the LORD your God will be with you wherever you go." Joshua 1:9 (NIV)

_____

_____

_____

_____

_____

_____

_____

_____

_____

_____

_____

_____

Conqueror's Notes

"Have I not commanded you? Be strong and courageous. Do not be terrified; do not be discouraged, for the LORD your God will be with you wherever you go." Joshua 1:9 (NIV)

_____

_____

_____

_____

_____

_____

_____

_____

_____

_____

_____

_____

_____

_____

Conqueror's Notes

"Have I not commanded you? Be strong and courageous. Do not be terrified; do not be discouraged, for the LORD your God will be with you wherever you go." Joshua 1:9 (NIV)

_____

_____

_____

_____

_____

_____

_____

_____

_____

_____

_____

_____

_____

_____

4

MEETING YOUR MEDICAL TEAM

S eptember 18, 2013 was my first medical visit for an initial consultation with a team of doctors, which consisted of my oncologist, Dr. Mahvish Muzaffar, surgeon Dr. James Wong and radiation oncologist Dr. Eleanor Harris at the Leo Jenkins Cancer Center in Greenville, NC. I knew that I was going to be receiving a lot of information from them, so I took a notebook with me to jot down information. I was so nervous when I arrived at the cancer center. I passed by the facility quite often, so I knew it was there and I had been there once many years ago with my mother, but now I was visiting it because I had become a patient. Walking through the doors and seeing people in wheelchairs, suffering from chemotherapy and its side effects was frightening for me. It was now surreal that I too would or could look and feel the same way. My husband Victor was right by my side, holding my hand, keeping me calm and my anxiety to a minimum. When you attend your first appointment or any appointment, take someone with you, so you can share your anxieties, fears and anxiousness. Just having someone there to talk to can help you keep things at a normalcy even though you are about to go through a rough time in your life.

Dr. Mahvish Muzaffar met with us and explained at length the stage of the cancer and how it would be beneficial to have preoperative chemotherapy, which would increase my chances of conserving the breast and my survival chances since it was found that I had triple negative breast cancer. According to the Susan G. Komen's website, hww5.komen.org, all breast cancer tumors are tested for certain receptors (proteins). These tests look for estrogen, progesterone and HER2/neu receptors. Test results are noted on a pathology report. If the tumors are "positive," there are many receptors. If the tumors are "negative," there are few or none. There are many treatment options for tumors that test "positive," but fewer options for those that do not. Triple negative breast cancer (TNBC) gets its name because the cells test negative for three receptors. So, TNBC is:

- Estrogen receptor-negative (ER-)

- Progesterone receptor-negative (PR-)

- HER2/neu-negative (HER2-)

TNBC is less likely to be found on a mammogram than some other types of breast cancer. It can also be aggressive. Compared to other types, it tends to grow faster. It can be treated, but it may come back early and spread to other parts of the body. Part of the reason is due to the lack of targeted treatments. Therefore, the chemotherapy chosen by Dr. Muzaffar would be aggressive and dense to ensure a modest impact on the cancer cells.

Knowing very little about the specifics of cancer, I learned my diagnosis of invasive breast cancer meant that it could invade nearby tissues, or enter the blood stream and lymphatic system, spreading to other organs. So, what are the stages of breast cancer and their meanings?

- **Stage 0:** This is *ductal carcinoma in situ (DCIS)*, a pre-cancer of the breast. Many consider DCIS the earliest form of breast cancer. In DCIS, cancer cells are still within a duct and have not spread.

- **Stage I:** The tumor is 2 centimeters or smaller and has not spread outside of the breast.

- **Stage IIA:** The tumor is still less than 2 centimeters, but the cancer has spread to the lymph nodes, which are located in the underarm area.

- **Stage IIB:** The tumor is larger than 5 centimeters, but no lymph nodes are affected. Or, the tumor is smaller than that, but cancer has spread to the lymph nodes.

- **Stage IIIA:** The tumor is smaller than 5 centimeters, but has spread to the lymph nodes. Or, it is larger than 5 centimeters, and has spread to the lymph nodes.

- **Stage IIIB:** The cancer has spread to the chest wall, skin or to the internal mammary lymph nodes on the same side of the chest.

- **Stage IV:** The cancer can be of any size and may or may not have spread to the lymph nodes. But it has spread to distant locations. According to research, the most common sites are the bones, liver, brain or lungs.

Please note that the staging of the cancer will be based on results of physical exam, biopsy, imaging tests like mammography and ultrasound, and the results of surgery. If you have any questions about the stage of your cancer, please be sure to ask your doctor.

During my visit with Dr. Muzaffar, I also met many wonderful nurses, one being a nurse navigator. She provided me with a plethora of information regarding breast cancer, treatments, nutrition and support. She assured me that anytime I had questions or concerns, she would be there to assist me. She was very kind and patient, with a sunny disposition. My fears and anxiety were slowly dissolving, as she and Dr. Muzaffar empowered my husband and I with more knowledge and understanding of the type of cancer I had and how they would be right there with me in the fight.

The second doctor working my case was Dr. Jan Wong, the surgeon who would be performing the surgery to remove the tumor. His specialty is surgical oncology. Before my visit, I thought that I would have the surgery first, then the chemotherapy and then the radiation. But because of the size of the tumor, it was recommended to have chemotherapy first. The breast would be left deformed and more than likely removed if not treated with chemotherapy. I wanted to conserve the breast if possible, but if it were required to be removed for survival, then it would have to go! To me, living was and is more important than having two breasts. I know many women who had their breast(s) removed and they are living productive lives, with one breast or no breasts. In addition to having the tumor removed, a lymph node in my left underarm would be removed as well to see whether the cancer had spread. I met his nurse and she made sure all my questions had been answered and if I understood the information given to me.

My final doctor would be Dr. Eleanor Harris, who specializes in radiation oncology and the physician in charge of my radiation treatments. Even though the treatments would not start until April 2014, she still met with me to introduce herself and explain the regimen, process and plan for treatments. I think I asked each doctor the very same question..." Do you think I will beat this?" And all of them told me that I could and would. No, I did not base my faith upon *their* answers or responses, but it sure did help me in those days to come when I did not think I could take another treatment, pill or hospital stay. It helped me through those days I looked in the mirror and didn't recognize myself and on those days, I didn't want anyone to see me.

If you meet your doctor(s) and you are not comfortable with what they are saying or do not understand any of the information, then ask questions and tell them that you do not understand. It is okay and their responsibility to listen to you and help you understand. If you find that you are not happy with what they are telling you or how you are being treated, then get yourself another doctor. Also, you may want to get a second opinion, which is your right as a patient. I was comfortable with my doctors and information received; therefore, I was not interested or felt the need for a second opinion.

For your convenience, here are some basic questions from the American Cancer Society's website, www.cancer.org that could help you talk to your doctor and start learning about the type of cancer you have and the choices you'll need to make.

- What kind of cancer do I have and what is my diagnosis?
- What is my cancer's stage and what does it mean for me?
- What are the benefits of my treatments?
- What are the risks?
- How soon do I need to start treatment?
- How long will I need treatment?
- What medicines will I get and what are they for?

- How should I expect to feel during treatment?
- What side effects can I expect to have?
- What can be done about the side effects?
- Can I work during treatment?

You do not have to become an expert about your condition; that's the doctor's job. But getting some of these questions answered will help you to be better prepared for what's ahead. And being informed helps you to make informed decisions. No one should make any decisions based on fear or assumption.

A Word of Encouragement

Currently Diagnosed – *Since your diagnosis, I am sure you have met with several doctors, nurses and possibly specialists. This can be overwhelming, but remember your medical team has your best interest at heart and want the very same thing you do; to become healthy again. They are working for you, so do not be afraid to ask questions or get a second opinion. This is your life and you only one to live!*

Conqueror – *It is beneficial to maintain a good relationship with your medical team, because they will continue to monitor your progress and ensure you remain healthy.*

Caregiver – *Whenever possible, accompany your loved one to the doctor. You would be amazed, as how much this will help them and you. This can be your opportunity to ask questions and obtain a better understanding of diagnosis, treatments, side effects, etc. Also, there may be bits of information your loved one may fail to disclose to the doctor and you can be there to help them remember, as well as obtain information once the appointment is over.*

Conqueror's Notes

My Medical Team

_____

_____

_____

_____

_____

_____

_____

_____

_____

_____

_____

_____

_____

Conqueror's Notes

My Medical Team

_____

_____

_____

_____

_____

_____

_____

_____

_____

_____

_____

_____

_____

_____

Conqueror's Notes

Important Telephone Numbers

_____

_____

_____

_____

_____

_____

_____

_____

_____

_____

_____

_____

_____

Conqueror's Notes

"Questions to Ask My Doctor"

_____

_____

_____

_____

_____

_____

_____

_____

_____

_____

_____

_____

Conqueror's Notes

"Questions to Ask My Doctor"

_____

_____

_____

_____

_____

_____

_____

_____

_____

_____

_____

_____

_____

5

PREPARING FOR CHEMOTHERAPY

*M*y oncologist informed me that I would be receiving my chemotherapy intravenously into my vein by a device called a port. The port was a small disc made of plastic about the size of a quarter that sits just under the skin. It would be surgically implanted in the right side of my chest. The procedure was simple and port was installed with no complications. It was completely under my skin and you could only see and feel a small bump on my chest. The use of the port prevented damage to my veins from the chemotherapy drugs and reduced the number of needle sticks to my very small veins.

The port installation was performed October 1st and my first chemo treatment was scheduled for October 9th. It was easy to take care of the port site and I did not experience any complications during installation or aftercare. A gauze dressing was placed over the site and home care instructions recommended it's changing every three days until my follow-up appointment. Also, a tub bath was preferred over a shower since I was supposed to keep the dressing dry. Wetness could cause an infection.

On my initial visit with the oncology team, the nurse navigator explained that I would experience hair loss two to four weeks after treatment due to the type of chemotherapy drugs I would receive. My regimen would consist of four treatments of ddAC every two weeks, followed by weekly Taxol for twelve weeks. Most women diagnosed with breast cancer, which has not spread to the lymph nodes, will receive this cocktail of drugs for treatment. I was not happy to hear that I would lose my hair, but I would rather lose my hair than to lose my life.

So, I decided that I would cut my short hair in preparation of it coming out. I hoped that I would be able to accept going from short hair to no hair than long hair to no hair/bald. I remember standing in front of my bathroom mirror with scissors cutting away my hair, my covering and my glory. I kept telling myself that it would grow back eventually. Once the mission was complete, I got in the shower to wash what hair I had left and broke down in tears. At that moment, it became more real to me that I had cancer and my anxiety went to another level. I have worn short hair before, but that was by choice. Here I was now with no choice in the matter and I would be completely bald. How could I be feminine or pretty with no hair? Yes, I was hurt and angry about it. But once I stopped having my pity party, I pulled myself together and again believed that this too would pass, with or without hair. And at the end of the day, if I truly wanted some hair, I could always go and buy some!

Every cancer patient does not choose chemotherapy as a part of his or her regimen. Some do not because of the harshness of the medications to the body. In my case, I was willing to do whatever I needed to do and chose to withstand the side effects of chemotherapy. My doctor recommended the treatment and I believed and trusted in her medical expertise. As you prepare yourself for chemotherapy and the possible loss of your hair, I have some great suggestions and knowledge of resources.

First, I was introduced to American Cancer Society McConnell-Raab Hope Lodge—Greenville, N.C. For those in need, they will give you a free wig, but it is on a first-come, first-serve basis. I could not find one that fit me or one that I preferred at the time, but at least there was a local place I could go and get one if I desired to do so. In the meantime, I decided to wear pretty scarves and fortunately, I had a few wigs already to wear. The scarves were more comfortable and fitting, so I wore those and make-up made me feel more feminine. Also, the Hope Lodge gave me a free make-up session with a make-up artist, who at the end of my session gave me a free make-up kit with lots of goodies. She was extremely nice and patient as she answered my questions, since I had little knowledge of some things, especially how to give myself eyebrows. They would fall out too so I wanted to be ready. And I did not want to walk around looking like I was surprised all the time or with two fuzzy caterpillars stuck on my face!

Second, another wonderful source is Mrs. Taushima Moore, owner and operator of Facets of Beauty Salon and Boutique, Inc. in Williamston, North Carolina. Mrs. Moore provides the service of customized wigs to anyone experiencing medical hair loss due to cancer treatments. To schedule a private consultation, which is free, you would call (252) 508-6691 or email her at facetsofbeautyinc@gmail.com. Before the consultation, here are a few things to consider:

1. **Figure out your budget.** Wigs range in price anywhere from $50 – thousands. In most cases, some insurance companies cover the cost (in part or completely).

2. **Determine what type of hair you want.**
   Generally, there are two types:
   > **Synthetic Hair.** This type of wig is
   made from strands that are created
   from polymers. Generally, synthetic
   wigs can hold a style through wear
   and shampoo. You must be careful,
   though because there are many types
   of synthetic wigs that cannot
   withstand high heat temperatures.
   Kanekalon is a type of synthetic hair
   that can be styled with a curling iron.

   > **Human Hair.** These wigs are made
   from real human hair or a mixture of
   human and animal that has been
   donated or sold to wig makers. These
   types of wigs can be colored, permed,
   cut, styled, and blow-dried, just like
   your own hair.

3. **Determine your look.** You can decide to
   keep the same hairstyle you had prior to
   losing your hair or be daring and try a totally
   fresh look. Maybe now is the time to try that
   look you have wanted to try for a while. At
   this point in your life, why not? Be

courageous, be bold and be daring! You deserve to look your best, so go for it.

For further information, please give Taushima a call. She would love to assist and give you one less thing to worry about while on your journey to wholeness.

And last but not the least, is Ms. Tia Johnson, owner and head stylist of Studio Adore' Mi on 4734D Reedy Branch Road in Winterville, North Carolina. Several women and I were blessed to be selected by Mr. Bobby Barnhill in 2013 to share our stories of overcoming adversity and we were awarded a free appointment at Ms. Johnson's salon and a photo shoot. Ms. Bernadine Cox assisted Mr. Barnhill with our photo shoot, making us feel like we were celebrities. It was a lot of fun and very relaxing; a time where I didn't have to think about cancer.

Ms. Johnson took such great care of us and made us look so beautiful that I began going to her salon for my hair appointments. When I lost my hair to chemo, Tia was so caring and compassionate. She made sure I was comfortable and ensured I had my privacy. For further information regarding her services or an appointment, please give Ms. Tia Johnson a call at (252) 258-7412.

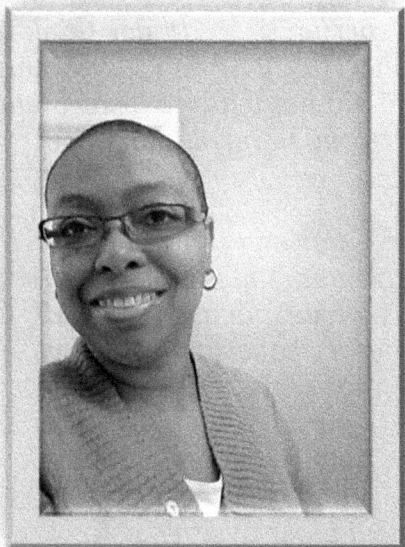

My New Hair Cut

Before Chemotherapy

October 7, 2013

A Word of Encouragement

Currently Diagnosed – *This can be an extremely traumatic experience, so do not think you are being vain. Do what fits you or makes you comfortable. Some days, I did not want to wear a wig, so I wore a pretty scarf or my natural, short hair.*

Conqueror – *For an extended period of time, I was uncomfortable with my natural hair, so I wore wigs. Recently, I received a haircut from Mrs. Silena Rascoe, owner and operator of Silena's House of Beauty and have been wearing my natural hair. With a mild texturizer and treatments, she has helped me maintain an easy and nice look, which I absolutely love! Her contact number is 252-522-5228; she would love to serve you.*

Caregiver – *Whatever makes your loved one comfortable, show your support and compliment them. You may not like the style or the look, but it wasn't your hair that fell out from the chemotherapy drugs. So, don't just like it, but love it!*

Conqueror's Notes

"And then he told me, "My grace is enough; it's all you need. My strength comes into its own in your weakness." Once I heard that, I was glad to let it happen. I quit focusing on the handicap and began appreciating the gift. It was a case of Christ's strength moving in on my weakness." 2 Corinthians 12:9 (MSG)

_____

_____

_____

_____

_____

_____

_____

_____

_____

_____

_____

_____

_____

Conqueror's Notes

"And then he told me, "My grace is enough; it's all you need. My strength comes into its own in your weakness." Once I heard that, I was glad to let it happen. I quit focusing on the handicap and began appreciating the gift. It was a case of Christ's strength moving in on my weakness." 2 Corinthians 12:9 (MSG)

_____

_____

_____

_____

_____

_____

_____

_____

_____

_____

_____

_____

Conqueror's Notes

"And then he told me, "My grace is enough; it's all you need. My strength comes into its own in your weakness." Once I heard that, I was glad to let it happen. I quit focusing on the handicap and began appreciating the gift. It was a case of Christ's strength moving in on my weakness." 2 Corinthians 12:9 (MSG)

_____

_____

_____

_____

_____

_____

_____

_____

_____

_____

_____

_____

_____

_____

_____

6

CHEMOTHERAPY DO'S & DON'TS

*I*t is common knowledge that many cancer patients do not take the route of chemotherapy, basically due to its side effects. I had heard many horrific stories of the nausea, vomiting and healthy cells being destroyed. But I also knew that my survival rate would decrease without it. Therefore, I decided to endure the side effects. Better yet, prayed to God that I would not be like the common case; but I would be the exception to the rule.

Before I get into this chapter's purpose, I want to share my first chemotherapy experience. My oncologist informed me that I would be receiving my first treatment on October 9th at 9:00AM. I would report to Leo Jenkins Cancer Center for lab work first (blood testing) and if my blood work was acceptable, I would then go over to Vidant Medical Center, 1 East for the intravenous treatment.

I would be there for several hours, so I took my iPad, a sweater and a blanket. My husband drove me to my appointment and I was glad that I didn't have to go alone. Just having him by my side made the time go by quicker and it was less scary having him with me. The nurses and caregivers were very compassionate and caring. The mood wasn't sad at all. Several patients who had been there before greeted one another and shared laughs and conversations with us newbies. Some patients slept through their treatments, while others read books, knitted, did puzzles or watched television.

For my first injection, I remember the nurse taking me to my reclining chair with awaiting monitors and empty poles for the IV bags. I noticed several televisions in each injection area for patients' convenience as well. As I sat down, I was greeted by an elderly lady who looked like she was in her eighties and was receiving medication. I spoke to her and settled down in the chair waiting to hear from nurse my next steps. While my heart raced from fear and anticipation, my husband and I attentively listened and watched the nurse as she prepped me for the chemotherapy drugs through the IV.

When the nurse stuck that needle into the port, which was under my skin, it hurt! I recommend that you purchase a lidocaine cream to numb the skin on top of the port for pain-free access to the port. Make sure you read the instructions because you need to give the medicine ample time to work. I also learned a trick of placing a big piece of saran wrap over the cream – it will help the skin absorb the lidocaine and keep it from rubbing off on your clothes until you get to the doctor's office or hospital for treatment. Honestly, sometimes the numbing medicine worked and there were some days it did not. On several occasions, the lab would be packed with blood work from awaiting patients. No one could receive their treatment unless their test results came back clear. So, during those times, the numbing medication would wear off.

As I received my medication, the elderly lady began to talk to me. I believe she could sense my anxiety and fear. She told me how she was in her eighties and even though she had cancer, she had no doubt that her faith would take her through it. She had been sick for a while and battled a lot of side effects from the medication, but each day she woke up, it was a blessing. With her sunny disposition, she assured me that I would be alright; just to keep trusting in Jesus. I thanked her for encouraging me and being such a light of hope. Sadly, I never saw her again, but I will always remember what she did for me that day.

Once my first treatment was completed, I was warned of the discoloration of my urine, but was told that it would eventually wear off once the drugs had worked their way out of my system. When it was time for me to go, I did feel a little woozy, but refused to be rolled out in a wheelchair. But if you feel the need to use one, please listen to your body; everyone reacts differently. My doctor warned me that I probably would not feel the effects of the chemotherapy until the next day, so just be prepared and take the prescribed anti-nausea medicine (*Dexamethasome*) well in advance. I felt fine, so I didn't take any, but drank plenty of water and rested the remainder of the day. Boy, I wished I had listened to the doctor. Don't go by how you feel; take the doctor's advice or pay for it later.

On the next day, I told my husband that he could go to work and I would be okay. He kept saying that he would stay home, but I urged him to go. He left for work, but made sure I had everything I needed. A couple of hours later, I felt this overwhelming nausea and sickening feeling. I got out of bed and began to look for the anti-nausea medication, but could not find it. It got so bad, that I crawled to the bathroom, anticipating violent vomiting. I could not stand up straight from feeling extremely dizzy and sick to my stomach. It was horrible! During this time, I could not call anybody; all I could do was pray and call on the name of Jesus. After vomiting in the bathroom, I crawled back to my bedroom to restart my search of the medication. I remembered that it was in my closet in one of my bags I had taken to the doctor. By the time I reached the closet, I was crying. Honestly, I was extremely upset with God because I felt He had ignored or denied my one request since being diagnosed with cancer. The request was that I not get sick in this manner and be able to go on and live a semi-normal life. I didn't think I was being selfish or unreasonable since the Scriptures say to ask what you will and just believe.

But here I was in my closet, crying, weak and unable to even stand up and get back on my bed. As I sat there, I cried out to God and I told Him that I didn't understand why He had allowed me to be sick in such an awful manner. I just knew that I would not have to take that medication and I would be one of those unaffected by the chemotherapy drugs. As I sat there sulking, trying to regain at least enough strength to climb back into bed, I heard the still voice of the Holy Spirit speaking these words to my heart and spirit, "The reason I allowed you to experience this is so that you would be able to appreciate all the other days that you wouldn't be sick." And it dawned on me of how could one appreciate health without the knowledge and experience of sickness? Or appreciate good times without knowledge and experience of the tough times? You can't! Immediately, I repented and told God that I was sorry for doubting that He knew what was best for me. Instead of complaining, I would be grateful for still being alive.

I finally found the anti-nausea medication in my bag and crawled back to the bed. Finally, able to climb back onto bed, which is high up off the floor, I downed the pills fast as I could. I knew it would take a while for me to feel any better, but I was grateful to have them in my system. I ate very little that day, mainly crackers and broth, but drank plenty of liquids, which I could keep down.

I must admit that I had several physical issues with chemotherapy, such as lack of appetite, taste changes, insomnia, hair loss, nails discoloration, mouth sores and fatigue. Therefore, I would like to make some suggestions to help you cope with the most worrisome side affects you may experience.

❖ **Lack of appetite (taste changes)** – with this side effect, my food started to have a metallic taste to it. All my favorite foods tasted weird or gave me severe indigestion, so I didn't want to eat.

> Do try new foods and recipes. Mexican food and green leafy vegetables were foods I could taste and would eat. My mother-in-law, Mother Jeanette Sheppard and friend Missionary Brenda Jenkins (a breast cancer conqueror) would cook kale for me. It tasted so good and was healthy for me. Another friend of mine, Missionary Rachel McCray cooked a green vegetable, I believe collards and gave me the liquid, which is called the pot liquor. I asked her for it and I drank it like a broth. It was filled with the vitamins and flavor of the greens. If the foods you decide to eat seem strange, don't worry about it. Whatever you can eat and keep down, eat it. Just make sure it is healthy. Other foods that I could eat were applesauce, bananas, rice and oatmeal.

> Do eat small meals or snacks whenever you can.
>   • At one point, I was hardly eating at all due to severe indigestion caused by the prescribed steroid, my anti-nausea medication. I started eating baby food because I just didn't know what to eat.

My husband would try to get me to eat but I didn't want to eat. If I did eat any regular food, I would have to sit up in the bed all night because of heartburn. One morning, my husband asked me if I wanted to go to the movies to get out of the house and I thought it was a great idea. I told him I would take a shower and get ready for the matinee. I got in the shower and surprisingly, started to sweat. I started feeling weird, so I decided to get out quickly. When I exited the shower, I yelled to my husband to bring me my bathrobe and that I was feeling funny. Well, after waking up on my bed nude, he explained to me that I had passed out in the bathroom as he entered with my bathrobe. Thank God, he caught me before I hit my head. When I awaken, he was on the phone with a 911 operator, explaining to them what had happened. There was one funny moment in this episode though. When I saw that I was naked on the bed, I looked up at my husband and said, "Hey I thought we were going to the movies! You got me up here all naked." He quickly hushed me since he was on the phone with the operator. He quickly dressed me and the EMT's arrived and drove me to the hospital. It was found that my lack of eating and the warm shower caused me to pass out. So, whenever you can, please eat.

➤ Don't eat fatty and fried foods. Baking or broiling your food is a better option.

➤ Drink plenty of liquids, especially water.

➤ Drink a nutritional drink like Ensure© or Boost© for vitamins and nutrients intake.

➤ Don't use metal utensils; use plastic ones, especially when you go out to eat. This will also help you with your defense against germs and keep the metallic taste to a minimum.

❖ **Mouth Sores** – Chemotherapy and radiation can cause mouth sores. Cancer treatments are intended to kill the rapidly growing bad cells, but some healthy cells will be damaged too. Also, chemo can impair your immune system, which fights off germs, viruses, bacteria and fungi. This can cause infections in the mouth, causing mouth sores. These sores can be very painful and make it hard to eat, and you may already be experiencing appetite issues. Therefore, here are some tips:

➤ See a dentist before starting treatments.

➤ Keep your mouth moist.

- Drink water and/or suck ice chips.

- Use sugar-free hard candy or gum.

- Use Biotin© mouthwash. This product helped me with dry mouth, which I still tend to still suffer from.

➤ Keep your mouth, tongue and gums clean.

- Don't use mouthwashes with alcohol in them. The alcohol will only cause you more pain and suffering.

- Brush your teeth with teeth, gums and tongue with an extra-soft toothbrush after every meal and at bedtime.

➤ Watch what you eat and drink.

- Try eating soft, moist foods like oatmeal, mashed potatoes and scrambled eggs.
- Choose foods that are easy to chew and swallow.

❖ **Insomnia** – I found myself sitting up all night at times, unable to go to sleep. The chemo had me tired and sleepy during the day, so I was up at night. Also, one of the side effects from my anti-nausea medicine was insomnia. Here are some suggestions:

➤ Take the supplement melatonin to help you fall asleep at night.

➤ Consume less amounts of caffeine and make sure you are not consuming them during the afternoon hours.

➤ Do something that relaxes you like listening to soothing music, reading or working on a quiet hobby such as crocheting, knitting or doing crossword puzzles.

➤ If you are prescribed a medication such as a steroid that interferes with your ability to sleep, speak with your doctor to see there is an alternative medicine. Also, you may want to take that medication early in the day and no later than 5:00PM or 6:00PM.

❖ **Neutropenia** – This is a condition when chemo has destroyed a high number of the neutrophils, which is a type of white blood cells. I was diagnosed with this on several occasions and my common symptom each time was a fever. You are more apt to catch an infection, when you are neutropenic. Therefore, during those times, I would have to wear a surgical mask when out in the public and could not eat any raw foods. It was also suggested to stay away from buffets due to the chance of easily catching germs. Even fresh flowers and anyone with a cold or flu were off limits.

➢ After my second chemo treatment, I had to return to the hospital to receive an injection of the drug, *Neulasta*, which stimulates the growth of white blood cells to help fight infection. My only side effect was bone pain, which wore off in a day or so. Before I was injected, I was warned that the medicine would have a burning

84

sensation as it went in. But it immediately wore off. I must admit though on the day after my Neulasta injection, I was getting out of my car and it felt like I had aged twenty years. Every bone in my body was aching! I took some ibuprofen and got some rest, which helped tremendously. On the market now is the Neulasta Onpro™ kit that includes a co-packaged single dose of Neulasta® and a single-use On-body injector, a small, lightweight delivery system applied to the skin during your chemo appointment. See the website for more information at www.neulasta.com.

❖ **Fatigue** – This is another common side effect of chemotherapy, but will vary person to person. It may come on suddenly and is not relieved by simply going to sleep or resting.

➢ Limit your activities. Decide what activities are important to you, and what could be delegated. Choose to use your energy on important jobs.

➢ Get plenty of rest. Balance between periods of rest and work. Pace yourself instead of sudden or lengthy tasks.

➢ Take vitamins or supplements if you are unable to maintain a healthy diet.

➢ Again, drink plenty of liquids. Most experts recommend a minimum of 8 cups of fluid per day, which will prevent dehydration. Fluids can include water, broth, milk, milkshakes and Jell-O.

❖ **Sensitivity to heat/sun** – This is an uncommon side effect of chemotherapy. I noticed after several treatments that I could not stand being in direct or indirect sunlight. Nor could I tolerate heat. If I exposed myself to heat or direct sunlight, my skin would start to feel as though thousands of pins were sticking in me. Then I would start to itch on my arms, legs, neck, face and back. It would become unbearable like a maddening itch and would continue until I cooled down. This side effect continued through my radiation treatments.

❖ **Depression** – I may have had one episode of helplessness and extreme sadness. I was headed to work one more and I wasn't feeling like myself. All I wanted to do was pull the covers over my head and stay in bed. I remember getting dressed and dragging myself to the car, only ending up crying in the car while driving to work. I drove about five miles and called my coworker Stacy House. I told her that I couldn't come to work like I had planned and I didn't know why I was feeling so hopeless. I was tired of the treatments, tired of feeling bad, tired of not looking like Lita, just tired of everything. She told me to go home and get some rest and that she would check on me later. She tried to encourage me, but I was not trying to hear it. As soon as I arrived back home, I cried out to God, praying that He would give me peace and take these feelings away. Five minutes later, my doorbell rang and it was another coworker Tiffany Wilson standing at the door. She told me that Stacy had called her and asked her to stop by and check on me. She attentively listened to me without judgment as I shared my heart and then she prayed for me. I gave her the biggest hug for just caring and taking the time to stop by and minister to me. I think both of us discovered some things about ourselves that day; I was not as strong as I thought I was and she *was* stronger than she thought she was.

Please keep in mind that side effects may differ from patient to patient. These are the ones I experienced. Another area of concern for me was sexual activity. I was worried about my husband being affected by the medicines I was taking at the time, but was assured by the doctor that there were no reasons to be concerned. If you feel well enough to have sex, then by all means, do it, but take precautions. Keep in mind chemotherapy can be excreted in vaginal secretions for 48-72 hours after a treatment. You should use a condom during this period to prevent your partner from being exposed to the chemotherapy. Also, if you have a low white blood cell count or low platelet count, you will need to refrain from any sexual activity that involves penetration. This is because there is an increased risk of infection or bleeding when your counts are low. But my best advice for everything is keeping communication open. Talk about what feels good and what doesn't; communicate with your partner when you are tired or uncomfortable.

From the chemotherapy treatments, I ended up in the hospital a few times. Two of my stays were for low white blood cells counts and fever. The longest hospital admission was four days in length and I had to have my port removed. I was tested for everything from MRSA to all infectious diseases and hooked up for intravenous antibiotics, fluids and blood transfusions. My husband was in the room with me one afternoon and in walks two doctors fully dressed in masks, protective clothing, gloves, goggles, etc. And we just looked at each other in amazement. My husband had on his normal street clothes and we were both thinking that I had the bubonic plague at this point. I asked them if they needed to tell us something like I was being quarantined for some infectious disease that could ruin mankind. But they assured us that they were only being cautious and following protocol.

While receiving shots daily in my stomach for blood clot prevention in my legs, some nights I was even hooked up to a cooling machine, which had cool water running through a pad that I laid on to bring the fever down. Nevertheless, nothing was found and after too many tests and needle poking's, it was finally determined that my port needed to be removed.

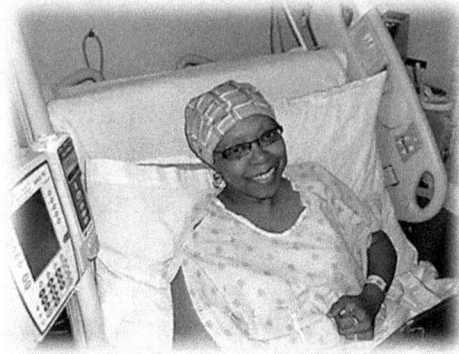

Once the port was removed, I did not experience any more fevers or hospital stays. I could go home one day after Christmas; disappointed that I had to spend Christmas in the hospital, but glad to be alive and was looking forward to the next Christmas.

On January 10, 2014, I experienced a miracle! Dr. Muzaffar walked in my examination room at one of my follow-up visits and told my husband and me that my chemotherapy treatments had been reduced from seven to two. Oh, my goodness! We were ecstatic and had to give God praise. Initially, I was scheduled for twelve (12) weekly treatments, which was reduced to only six! Even though my port was removed, I only had two more treatments of chemotherapy and would not have to worry about the effects of chemotherapy to my veins.

I was fortunate to get through those last two treatments without the use of a port and any complications. My veins were very small, but each time, one was used in my hand. Some patients keep their ports in even after treatments are completed, for blood withdrawals. I am glad mine was removed; the bump under my skin was a constant reminder of cancer and what I had gone through. No, the removal does not completely wipe away all the memories of it. Besides, I have a small scar where the port once resided, but at least all it is now is a memory of being more than a conqueror, not just a survivor or victim of cancer.

My last chemotherapy treatment was February 14, 2014, Valentine's Day. Now how sweet was that? I made a sign to celebrate that special day and my husband took a picture of me with some of the wonderful nurses who had taken care of me during my treatments. What an awesome way to memorialize that moment and an extremely special Valentine's Day.

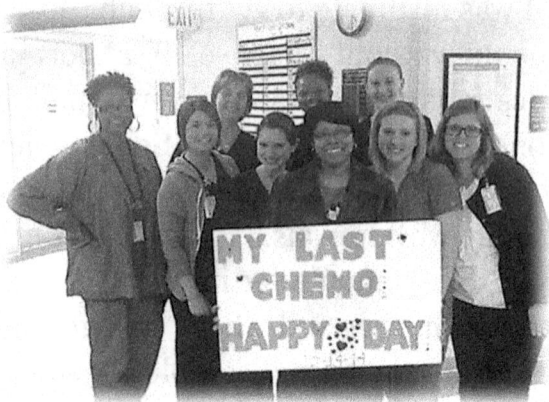

Nurses at 1 East Vidant Medical Center
February 14, 2014

Celebrate your victories, no matter how small you may think it is. Remember, you deserve it and each step closer to wellness is reason for celebration and rejoicing. It's just our way of showing cancer who's boss!

A Word of Encouragement

Currently Diagnosed – *Ask your oncologist/nurse navigator lots of questions. Prepare yourself physically, mentally & spiritually for this part of your journey. I cannot promise you that it will be easy. But what I can say, is that through God, I showed cancer who was boss and you can too!*

Conqueror – *As a Conqueror, you know that it was not a walk in the park, but you overcame it. With that same tenacity, you can overcome anything you may be facing. Never give up! God's grace is still sufficient.*

Caregiver – *This time can be extremely painful for you as you watch your loved one experience the horrible side effects of chemotherapy. Whenever you are able, please take time to take care of you. If you are accompanying them to their treatments or having to take care of them around the clock, ask another family member to help so you can get away for a while. This will not only help you, but your loved one as well.*

Conqueror's Notes

"So, we're not giving up. How could we! Even though on the outside it often looks like things are falling apart on us, on the inside, where God is making new life, not a day goes by without his unfolding grace." *2 Corinthians 4:16 (MSG)*

_____

_____

_____

_____

_____

_____

_____

_____

_____

_____

_____

_____

Conqueror's Notes

"So, we're not giving up. How could we! Even though on the outside it often looks like things are falling apart on us, on the inside, where God is making new life, not a day goes by without his unfolding grace." 2 Corinthians 4:16 (MSG)

_____

_____

_____

_____

_____

_____

_____

_____

_____

_____

_____

_____

Conqueror's Notes

"So, we're not giving up. How could we! Even though on the outside it often looks like things are falling apart on us, on the inside, where God is making new life, not a day goes by without his unfolding grace." 2 Corinthians 4:16 (MSG)

_____

_____

_____

_____

_____

_____

_____

_____

_____

_____

_____

_____

_____

7

SURGERY

*D*uring my bout with cancer, I had a total of three surgeries. Two were the installation and removal of the port. And the third surgery was the lumpectomy and removal of one lymph node, which occurred on March 13, 2014. The lumpectomy was performed after the tumor was treated with chemotherapy to shrink it. Also, the tissue around the lump was removed and the one lymph node.

My port was installed a few days before my first chemotherapy treatment. I thought since it was surgery even though categorized as being minor, I would still be put to sleep. Wrong! I kept waiting for the doctor to give me the anesthesia, but it never happened. I even asked the attending nurse because I was getting worried. I did not want to feel any pain if necessary. She calmly noted that it was not needed, but the area would be numbed to where I would not feel any pain or discomfort. I thought to myself, "Well that's easy for you to say. You're not the one being cut!" Nevertheless, the area was numbed completely and port installed. It only took about fifteen minutes, which was fast! Keep in mind that medical professionals do these types of procedures on a daily basis and some may not take into consideration that you may be uneasy or afraid. I have experienced a few bedside manners which were cold and unfriendly; very direct and to the point. But in the end, they did their job and did it well. Some things you will have to take with a grain of salt, and not take it personal.

One of my questions for my surgeon at my initial visit with him was why chemotherapy before the tumor's removal. Shrinking the tumor before surgery was for the conservation of my breast and to leave it in its normal state. Removing the tumor at its initial size would have caused my breast to look abnormal and the whole breast would have needed to be removed. When that type of procedure is necessary, it is called a mastectomy. But the removal of one of my lymph nodes was done to test it to see if the cancer had spread. When my results came back, I was given great news; the cancer had not spread! Thank you, Jesus, which it was caught in time and all the cancer was removed.

The only complication I had during this surgery was my blood pressure dropping too low. Of course, I wasn't aware of this since I was out cold, but when I awaken, my husband Victor was right by my side and explained it to me while I was in recovery. We both were grateful that once again, God had blessed me to leap another hurdle in my race to wellness.

Depending on the size of the tumor and stage of cancer, the doctor will decide on the best time of its removal. I could return home on the same day after the outpatient procedure was done at Vidant Medical Center. Generally, if a mastectomy is performed then a one-night hospital stay is the normal protocol. Also, keep in mind that a lumpectomy and radiation treatments are a packaged deal. Not having radiation can increase your chances of the cancer coming back. And who wants or needs that?

Before the lumpectomy was performed, I had a wire localization done by radiology. The clip allowed accurate localization or position of the tumor's site for removal, so that as little tissue as necessary was removed. And to boost the chances of clear margins, meaning getting all the cancer cells removed.

At the clip's installation procedure, I was given a mammogram and shown just how much the tumor had shrunk after being treated with chemotherapy. I was amazed and thrilled to know that the treatments had worked! I wanted to keep the X-ray, but they wouldn't let me. If I had been thinking clearly, I would have taken a picture of it with my cell phone. Nevertheless, the image is etched into my memory and truly it was a moment of joy to see that the pain and discomfort was well worth it.

As I mentioned before, my last surgery was the removal of the chemotherapy port. After the attending doctors had ruled out infectious diseases, it was suggested to remove it. The procedure was just as quick as the installation; and I could go home after being in the hospital over the Christmas holiday. Sadly, I even missed my daughter's engagement proposal. I knew it was an extremely special moment for her and encouraged her fiancé, now my son-in-law, to go ahead with his plans. And I did not want him to do it at the hospital either. I chose to believe that we would have plenty of time to celebrate and make better memories than what we were going through at the time.

Regarding a mastectomy, please seek information and advice from your doctor regarding this procedure. Since I did not undergo that procedure, I prefer not to offer information. But, here are more suggestions and information regarding a lumpectomy.

❖ Lymph Node(s) Removal – As I mentioned earlier, I only had one removed. But there are cases in which a patient may need several removed. And in these instances, removing several lymph nodes can lead to complications in the area such as fluid buildup which is called lymphedema. Lymphedema is a build-up of lymph fluid in the fatty tissues just under the skin. Fortunately, I did not experience it. But a friend of mine did. She had to wear the compression sleeve and noted how painful it could be.

➤ What causes it?

▪ When lymph nodes are removed, vessels that carry fluid from the arm to the rest of the body are also removed. The removal changes the flow of the lymph fluid and with breast cancer, it makes it harder for fluid in the chest, breast, and arm to flow out of these areas. If the fluid is not drained enough from these areas, the fluid builds up and causes swelling or lymphedema.

- Lymphedema can start soon after surgery and/or radiation treatment. Mostly it develops slowly over time. But it can also start months or even many years later.

➤ What to do after surgery or radiation to help reduce swelling?

- Use your affected arm as you normally would when combing your hair, bathing, dressing, and eating.

- Put your affected arm above the level of your heart 2 or 3 times a day and keep it there for 45 minutes. Lie down to do this, and fully support your arm. Place your arm up on pillows so that your hand is higher than your wrist and your elbow is a little higher than your shoulder.

- Exercise your affected arm while it's supported above the

level of your heart by opening and closing your hand 15 to 25 times. Repeat this 3 to 4 times a day. This helps reduce swelling by pumping lymph fluid out of your arm through the undamaged lymph vessels.

- Avoid anything tight around the arm (like a tourniquet used to draw blood, a blood pressure cuff, or a tight band on a sleeve) on the affected side.

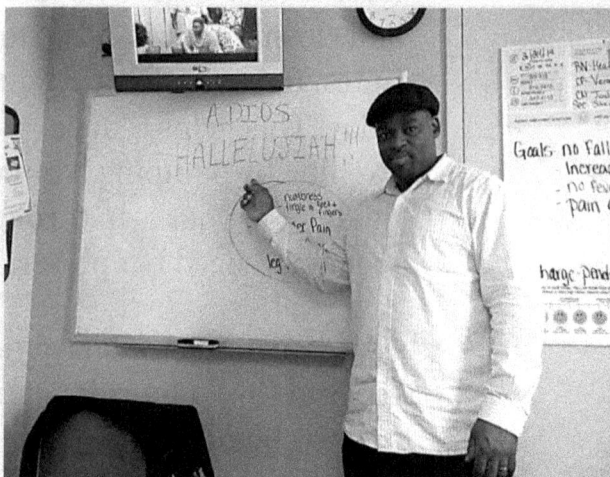

My Husband Victor Celebrating My Last Day in Hospital over the Holidays December 27, 2013

A Word of Encouragement

Currently Diagnosed – *Any type of surgery can be scary. So, share your fears with support team and doctors. But if your doctor prescribes it, take courage in knowing that it is just one step closer to being whole again. If that means having your breast remove, please understand that no body part makes you who you are. It is your heart that matters!*

Conqueror – *Do you still have scars (physical or mental) that you are still dealing with or feel* *uncomfortable about? I used to be very conscientious about mine, but now, I see them as battle scars and badges of courage. They remind me of where I have been, and with God's grace, what I have conquered.*

Caregiver – *If you are present for surgical procedures or appointments, help your loved one to ask questions regarding complications, aftercare and medications. Get as much information you can to assist in their care at home. It will make your life easier and put their mind at more ease.*

Conqueror's Notes

"Don't fret or worry. Instead of worrying, pray. Let petitions and praises shape your worries into prayers, letting God know your concerns." Philippians 4:6 (MSG)

_____

_____

_____

_____

_____

_____

_____

_____

_____

_____

_____

_____

Conqueror's Notes

"Don't fret or worry. Instead of worrying, pray. Let petitions and praises shape your worries into prayers, letting God know your concerns." Philippians 4:6 (MSG)

_____

_____

_____

_____

_____

_____

_____

_____

_____

_____

_____

_____

Conqueror's Notes

"Don't fret or worry. Instead of worrying, pray. Let petitions and praises shape your worries into prayers, letting God know your concerns." Philippians 4:6 (MSG)

_____

_____

_____

_____

_____

_____

_____

_____

_____

_____

_____

_____

8

RADIATION TREATMENTS

*a*ccording to breastcancer.org, most people receive 5 to 7 weeks of radiation therapy shortly after lumpectomy to eliminate any cancer cells that may be present in the remaining breast tissue. The combination of lumpectomy and radiation therapy is commonly called breast-conserving therapy. If chemotherapy is also part of the plan, radiation therapy happens after chemotherapy and a lumpectomy.

Before receiving my radiation treatments, I went in and the radiation therapist did a "simulation", which marked the exact spot where I would receive radiation. It was explained that several scans would be performed and then with a marker, they would mark the areas on my body to receive radiation. It was also explained that I could opt to have small tattoo dots placed on the areas to be treated, so I would not have to be "marked" with a pen/marker each time I came to be treated. Well, I am a big girl and quite frankly, I had been curious of how it felt to get a tattoo. So, I told the therapist I wanted to try the tattoo dot, but was afraid of the pain. So, she explained that she would do a small test dot in the middle of my chest.

Oh, my goodness! When she stuck that needle in my chest, I almost jumped off the examination table! I quickly told her, "Ma'am, ple-e-e-e-ease use the marker and write on me all you want to! Draw pictures if you feel like!" No needles or tattoos for this girl! I still have the tiny needle prick to remind me of it and that will be the only tattoo on this body. I have a high tolerance for pain, but I guess not for that.

My radiation regimen was five days a week for six weeks, plus seven boost treatments. The boosts were in a more concentrated section than the entire treated area, targeting the tumor bed, which was in my armpit or under my arm. I scheduled the treatments in the afternoons so I could work in the morning; go for treatments in the afternoon and then home to rest. Each time I went to get my treatment, I knew I was one step closer to being done. Many times, I would be in the lobby or in the pre-treatment area waiting to be called back, and I would see a patient being brought in on a hospital or ambulatory bed. They were too weak or sick to walk in on their own. My heart would grieve for them and their family, and I would tell myself to stop complaining and be thankful. I could drive myself to and from these appointments, so I did not have any right or reason to moan and groan. Life has a way of shaking and reminding you that things could be so much worse.

I received my first treatment April 28, 2014 and the treatments only lasted for about fifteen minutes. The medical staff would play any genre of music per my request and while lying on the exam table flat on my back, I would hum to the music, recite my favorite Scriptures and pretend I was somewhere else. I welcomed the music in hopes that it would drown out the humming sound of the radiation machine. Hearing it only made me think of a laser beam shooting at me. I know it may sound silly, but this huge machine sending radiation inside my body was not a picnic or day at the park. It still was a little scary, but a lot better than the chemotherapy.

One wonderful thing about the examination room was that its ceiling was made partly of glass, so I could see the sunshine. Often, I would pretend that I was lying on the beach without a care in the world. Other times I would take that moment to meditate and pray in my heart that God was using this time to heal me and make me rest. Every now and then, I would hear the loud bumping and knocking of the machine, which would only bring me back to the reality of where I actually was.

The main side effects I experienced were fatigue and skin irritations. The actual treatment was not painful, but as my underarm skin received more radiation, the more tender and painful that area of my body became. Truthfully, I thought that my skin in my armpit was going to tear. The skin in that area was extremely thin and the concentrated boost treatments were targeted right on it. I was so worried that the skin would tear, and my treatments would have to be postponed. But, thankfully it didn't happen.

I did experience extreme itching whenever I was in direct sunlight or became too hot. It felt like a prickling of my skin, as if someone was sticking small needles in me. Then I would start itching like I had hives. It would become unbearable and I would not go outside for days on end due to the fear of having these episodes. And it did not just happen from being outside, but if I got too hot while inside, it would happen as well.

Here are some recommendations:

❖ Wear loose, soft clothing, preferably cotton that is less irritating to the affected area.

❖ Avoid direct exposure to sunlight. Protect the area from the sun.

❖ When bathing, use a mild soap and warm water.

❖ Moisturize your skin with Aquafor© or Eucerin©, which can be purchased over-the-counter at your local Wal-Mart or drugstore. I used Aquafor© on my skin while taking chemotherapy treatments as well. It helped with the dry skin and irritations.

  ➢ The skin receiving radiation darkened in color and became drier and flaky. The moisturizer helped the dryness and minimized the irritation. My breast is still darker than the other one and has not returned to its original pigment.

But after almost two months of radiation treatments, my last radiation treatment was June 13, 2014. In the lobby of the Leo Jenkins' Cancer Center, the Bell of Hope hangs on the wall for patients who are receiving their last radiation or chemotherapy treatment. Once you complete that final treatment, you are handed a small metal mallet and you hit that bell with great intensity or absolute frenzy. Hitting that bell says, "I made it! It may have been a struggle, but I did more than just survive. I conquered cancer! Now I can celebrate another victory of life! I will not live in fear! I will finish the fight until the very end by showing cancer who's boss!"

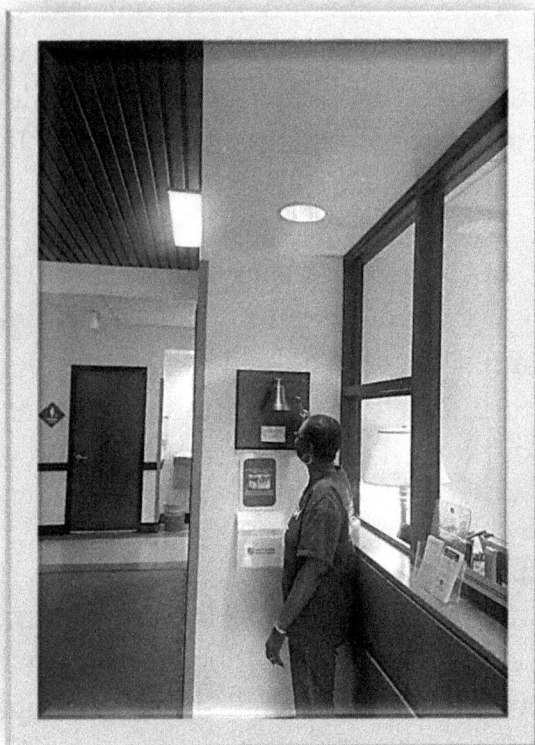

Ringing the Hope Bell at Leo Jenkins Cancer Center

June 13, 2014

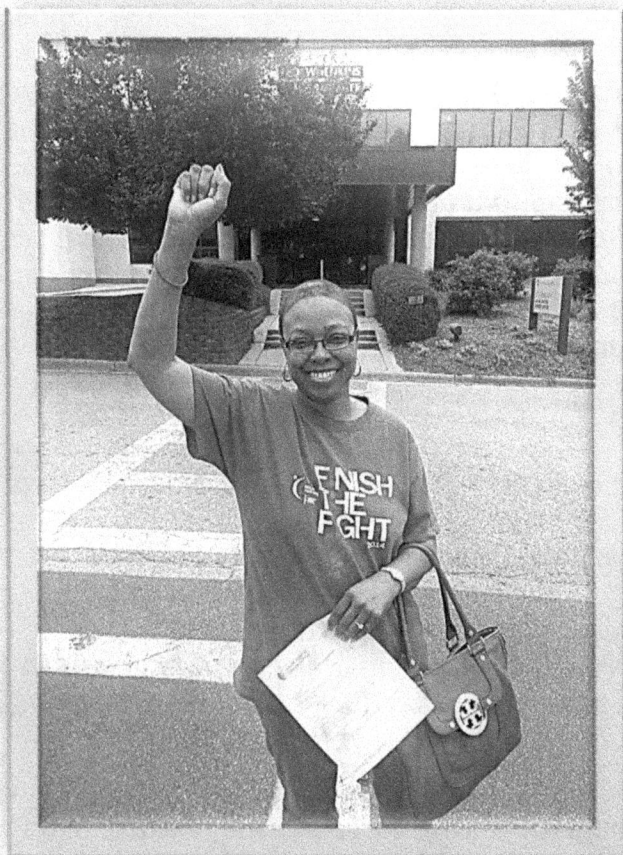

**Celebrating My Last Radiation
Treatment in Front of Leo Jenkins
Cancer Center**

June 13, 2014

A Word of Encouragement

Currently Diagnosed – *It is my prayer that once you get to this stage, you will be almost done with your cancer treatments. When I had the lumpectomy, I was told that the cancer had been removed. And the radiation was just to ensure that no cancer cells remained. I don't think that it registered in my brain that technically, I was cancer-free after surgery. So, when the time comes for you, C-E-L-E-B-R-A-T-E! You deserve it!*

Conqueror – *Do you remember your last treatment or last visit? Sheer jubilation, right? Yeah, I was too; as you can see in my picture. But I also can attest to the low energy and emotional moments you may be experiencing. Remember that it is in your rear-view mirror; look ahead and take one day at a time. Rest when necessary, but do not stay there too long. You still have a lot of life left to live.*

Caregiver – *Your loved one may be able to transport themselves back and forth to treatments, but at least offer your time and assistance. Some days, they may not feel up to par and a little help would be greatly appreciated. And if they do not want the help, just be watchful in case you need to step in and make them accept your help.*

Conqueror's Notes

"He gives power to the weak and strength to the powerless. Even youths will become weak and tired, and young men will fall in exhaustion. But those who trust in the LORD will find new strength. They will soar high on wings like eagles. They will run and not grow weary. They will walk and not faint."
Isaiah 40:29-31 (NLT)

Conqueror's Notes

"He gives power to the weak and strength to the powerless. Even youths will become weak and tired, and young men will fall in exhaustion. But those who trust in the LORD will find new strength. They will soar high on wings like eagles. They will run and not grow weary. They will walk and not faint."

Isaiah 40:29-31 (NLT)

_____

_____

_____

_____

_____

_____

_____

_____

_____

_____

_____

_____

Conqueror's Notes

*"He gives power to the weak and strength to the powerless.
Even youths will become weak and tired, and young men will
fall in exhaustion. But those who trust in the LORD will find
new strength. They will soar high on wings like eagles. They
will run and not grow weary. They will walk and not faint."*
Isaiah 40:29-31 (NLT)

_____

_____

_____

_____

_____

_____

_____

_____

_____

_____

_____

9

THE IN BETWEENS

This chapter almost didn't make the final cut of writing this book. I was so excited about finishing the book, I almost omitted a very important part of survivorship; what to do in between the different phases of your journey to wellness. Activities, moments, events, days, weeks, months and years will not and cannot be identical for any two people. You may be experiencing some ailments or damages from the chemotherapy that I was fortunate not to have experienced. But the purpose of this chapter is to inspire and motivate you to keep moving and do whatever you can while you are in between your healing and wholeness.

If there are days you can work, then go to work and grab those moments of getting back to normal. There were days I didn't feel up to going to work, but I went anyway. When my immune system was compromising and more receptive to germs, I wore a face mask. I refused to allow my pain, discomfort or anything to hold me hostage. Just the feeling of the sunshine or wind on my face was a reminder that I was still alive and anything was possible. I was determined to push and not allow my condition to keep me down. When it is possible, try to obtain some normalcy in your life. My mother-in-law, Mrs. Jeanette Sheppard would drive over to my house routinely to check on me, but on most days, I would be out of the house. She would call me in her concerned voice, saying, "Daughter, where are you at now? You better get back in that house and rest!" We would laugh, I'd tell her my whereabouts and ask her to not call and tell Mickey (my husband's nickname). I would ensure her that I would get back home in a reasonable amount of time though.

Many times, I pushed myself to get out of the house; one being to accompany my husband to one of our grandson's, Jamarion baseball games. I didn't feel my best, but after going, I felt better. When you get into the routine of being sedentary or stuck in the house, it is hard to break out of that mold. But you must get moving again. An active lifestyle will help you physically and mentally. According to the American Cancer Society, obesity (being very overweight), is linked to a higher risk of many types of cancer, a higher risk of certain cancers coming back after treatment, and worse survival for many types of cancer.

Your family can play a very important role in support at this stage as well. My husband, children, sisters and mothers threw me a Surprise

50th birthday party. What an awesome time I had with family and friends, enjoying old memories and making new ones! There were lots of great food (crab legs and my pastor's wife's famous macaroni and cheese), music and laughter. It wasn't just a day of celebrating my birthday, but a celebration of overcoming and looking forward to the future. In between radiation treatments, I was a bridesmaid in my husband's cousin's wedding party. Here was another beautiful memory to cherish and be a part of as Jeff and Twebe Ward committed a lifetime of love to each other in the presence of family and friends.

Initially for the wedding, I was worried about my hair being short and the surgical scars showing in the pictures due to the bridesmaid dresses' style. Then it hit me! I realized I could have been dead and instead of participating in a wedding, I could have been the guest of honor at my own funeral. I got over the worrying of my looks rather quickly and had a wonderful time. I was so thankful to be able to enjoy this wonderful occasion and help them celebrate their wedding.

Once you are feeling more and more like yourself, you may want to volunteer with cancer-related organizations, events or maybe in another area of interest. At this point, you can use your experience to help someone else, even if it is just to listen and acknowledge someone's concerns or fears. I have learned that our tests become testimonies to share with others and help them to overcome as we have. God does not waste any experiences in our lives. Galatians 3:4 asks the question whether we have suffered in vain. And my reply is no! Not only have I learned invaluable lessons about myself, but about my relationship with God and others. This in turn has made me better, not bitter and not broken.

As you go through your journey, many discoveries will be made about yourself; some areas requiring improvement, like your attitude and spiritual belief system. The area of attitude would be how you think or perceive things; whether your response, reaction or behavior is positive or negative. My spiritual belief system is CHRISTianity; characteristically based more on relationship than religious practices. It is not just something I do, but more of what Jesus Christ did for me. And now, because of His love and compassion for me, I want to share that with others. My cancer experience has presented me with many gifts; gifts of sharing my experience through this guidebook, talking with people about how to live beyond cancer, and a new lease on life and love.

124

The in between stage is not only to show cancer who's boss, but to show you that you are a lot stronger than what you thought and there is a lot more to life to be lived intentionally. If you have made it this far, you can still go a little further. You have enough strength and resilience to take another step; get up out of that bed or chair, live life and love harder!

My 50th Birthday Celebration

May 27, 2014

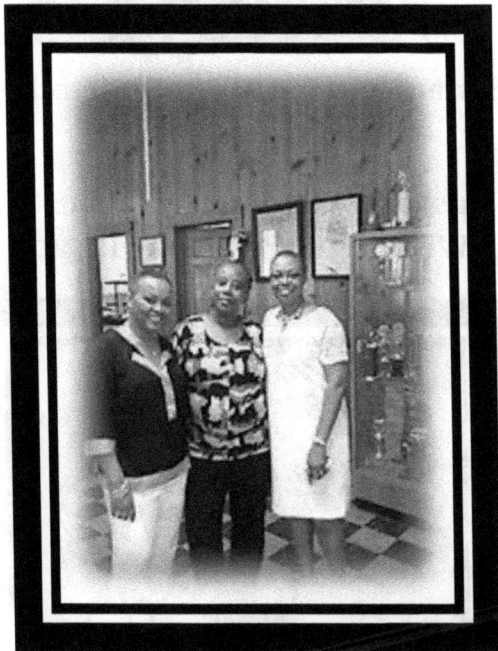

**God Daughter Lakita Corey
and First Lady Deloris Wilkins**

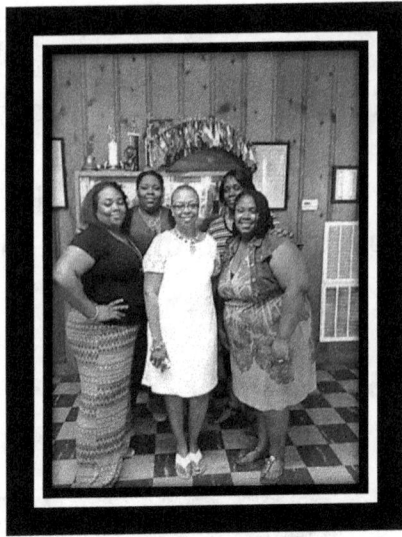

My Sisters and I at My 50th Birthday Party

My Husband Victor and I in our Cousin's Wedding Party – July 12, 2014

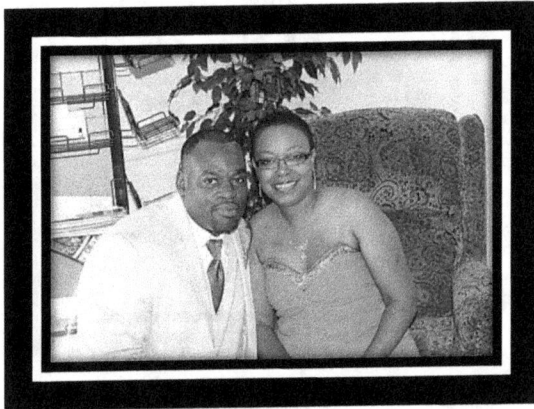

A Word of Encouragement

Currently Diagnosed – *Hold on to your faith! You will get to this point and be able to look back in amazement of the remarkable things you have learned during your journey to now.*

Conqueror – *If you are here in this moment, take a moment and think about all of things you have learned. Also, ask yourself, "What am I doing to help someone else who may be experiencing what I have already?" Use this time as a moment of discovery and/or motivation to do more with your gifts.*

Caregiver – *Use this time as a way to get your loved one back out in the world through simple activities. A walk in the park or neighborhood; having lunch or dinner together would help change the scenery. Any type of activity for normalcy would be great to help get your loved one back in flow of things.*

Conqueror's Notes

"You have turned my mourning into joyful dancing.
You have taken away my clothes of mourning and clothed me
with joy, that I might sing praises to you and not be silent.
O Lord my God, I will give you thanks forever!"
Psalm 30:11-12 (NLT)

_____

_____

_____

_____

_____

_____

_____

_____

_____

_____

_____

Conqueror's Notes

"You have turned my mourning into joyful dancing.
You have taken away my clothes of mourning and clothed me
with joy, that I might sing praises to you and not be silent.
O Lord my God, I will give you thanks forever!"
Psalm 30:11-12 (NLT)

_____

_____

_____

_____

_____

_____

_____

_____

_____

_____

_____

Conqueror's Notes

*"You have turned my mourning into joyful dancing.
You have taken away my clothes of mourning and clothed me
with joy, that I might sing praises to you and not be silent.
O Lord my God, I will give you thanks forever!"*
Psalm 30:11-12 (NLT)

_____

_____

_____

_____

_____

_____

_____

_____

_____

_____

_____

_____

10

NOW WHAT?

*M*any have the preconception that once a cancer patient is in remission, it is life back to usual or normal. Unfortunately, that is far from the truth. I am now more conscious of making better food choices, being more active, having a more intimate relationship with God, my family and worrying less about those things I cannot change.

The frequency of my doctor's appointments decreased, but I remain in contact with my doctors and nurse practitioner, Elizabeth Gottsch. Elizabeth would see me on my follow-up visits and always there to answer my questions. Always attend your doctor's appointments. It is extremely important for you to remain on schedule with your preventive care.

I was placed on the breast cancer drug called Anastrozole (Arimidex®), which I take one pill daily. Because I was postmenopausal, it was prescribed to reduce the risk of the cancer coming back and lower my estrogen hormone levels. With any or most medications, there will be side effects.

131

For me, I have hot flashes, vaginal dryness, hair thinning, tiredness and some bone pain. And in all fairness, these symptoms occur from menopause as well.

But to monitor my heart function and bone density, I have had echocardiograms and bone density tests performed. The echo examination showed no damage to my heart from chemo, but I have quite a bit of bone loss, meaning I am more apt to have osteoporosis. This bone disease develops when the body breaks down more bone tissue than it can replace. As a result, bones become weak and fragile, making them more likely to fracture or break. My oncologist prescribed calcium and vitamin D supplements. The current recommendations are listed below. Before **you** take any vitamin or mineral supplement, talk with your doctor.

> Vitamin D: 800 international units (IU) per day for women of all ages
> Calcium supplements for women before menopause: 1,000 milligrams (mg) per day
> Calcium supplements for women after menopause: 1,200 mg per day

Also, exercising was recommended. Weight-bearing physical activities such as walking, dancing, and stair-climbing put stress on your bones. This stress triggers the body to make cells that form bone. Regular weight-bearing exercise also builds strong muscles, which can help your balance. Your doctor can recommend an exercise plan based on your needs, physical abilities, and fitness level.

Finally, I was told to consider the bone medication *Denosumab* to lower the amount of calcium loss from bone and to treat osteoporosis. These medications would be administered annually at my local hospital and the side effects read quite like the milder symptoms of chemo medications. Ironically, my 71-year-old mother has recently been placed on the same regimen of calcium and vitamin D supplements intake, plus the annual injection. I guess the chemo helped my bones age almost 20 years.

The hot flashes have become almost non-existent, but the vaginal dryness can be extremely painful. This will even warrant low libido because it hurt so badly. Thankfully, there are over-the-counter products which work quite effectively. I recommend *Replens Long-lasting Vaginal Moisturizer©* and an open discussion with your partner. If he is aware of what you are experiencing, then he will be more understanding and caring. I use the *Replens* every three days and it helps tremendously. Also, you could use a lubricant, which will work as well. You would just have to use that each time before you are intimate.

Nevertheless, don't live your life in fear of reoccurrence. Yes, I think about often, sometimes too much. As a matter of fact, just a few days ago, I was getting ready for bed, and I thought I felt a knot in my chest. "Lord; please not again!" I thought to myself. I kept pressing on it and fearing for the worse. I went to bed that night, but did not drift off to sleep until around 1:00AM. As soon as the doctor's office opened, I called them asking if I could leave a message for the nurse to call me about this discovery. Well, after calling them, I ran an errand and drove straight to the office. I explained my fear to the receptionist and she found the nurse for me, who took me to an examination room. She explained that my surgeon was in a conference, but would be right over to check me out. The wait seemed like forever, even though it was only thirty minutes.

When Dr. Wong arrived, he examined me and said that he did not feel anything that resembled a lump. I was relieved, but he could tell that I was still worried. He calmly patted my hand and said, "Don't worry; you are okay. There's nothing there to be worried about." At that moment, I was reminded that **F.E.A.R.** was nothing more than "**F**alse **E**vidence **A**ppearing to be **R**eal."

Even my husband tells me all the time, to not think about so much. But that is easier said than done. So instead of allowing it to be a negative, I choose to turn it into a positive. How you may ask? It is a constant reminder to make better use of my time and life. One minute everything was going well, and wham! Out of nowhere, I had stage 3 cancer. In the world we live in, nothing seems to be constant and unchanging. But the love of Christ and His Word never changes and is a constant reminder that if you just keep the faith and trust in Him, everything will work out. Even though I have some physical challenges, I still keep it moving. Having another chance at life should motivate you to get it right this time. What is my "it"? It is my relationships, purpose, goals, visions and dreams. Focus more on those things and less on thoughts of what if *it* comes back. Always be hopeful and live your life to the fullest!

In your local community or online, you can easily find support groups to join or become a part of. This may or may not be for you and either way, it is okay. Personally, I have joined online support groups because of my work schedule and busy personal life. From to time, I take off and attend workshops offered by Leo Jenkins Cancer Center and the American Cancer Society. It can be extremely helpful and relieving to be able to share your experiences and hear others tell theirs. You would be amazed to hear the commonalities and things they have found helpful.

As of today, I have successfully published three books, which includes this one and travel across the state motivating and empowering people to pursue their purpose. Also, I stepped into the arena of entrepreneurship by starting LPW Editing and Consulting Services and I have been blessed to partner with Cannon Publishing as their chief editor. None of these accomplishments occurred because I was smart, wealthy or wise; but I made conscious decisions to walk in purpose by using my God-given gifts and abilities.

If you have picked up this book and cancer has reoccurred or advanced in your body or someone you love, *do not give up*! It is my goal to share my story to inspire and prove that cancer is no longer a death sentence, but something that comes to test your will to live and to not just survive, but thrive. You will probably experience many different emotions such as anger, grief or despair, which would be normal reactions. But you cannot stop there and remain there. Express your emotions and share your fears, but *do not give up and do not stop fighting*! I know several women who have experienced reoccurrences and one thing they did not do was give up or give in. So, neither should you or your loved one.

No one knows or can predict accurately when and if cancer will return; sometimes even the cause of it. Because I was not a smoker or drinker, my doctor asked me if I wanted to have a genetic test performed to see if I had the BRCA1 or BRCA2 genes. Mutations can be passed to you from either parent and can affect the risk of cancers in both women and men. I agreed to the test because I wanted to know whether my daughter or sons were at risk. My results were inconclusive and those cancer-causing genes were not found.

But what one thing I can be certain of is that a meaningful life is not based on quantity (number of years) but quality (Whose life did you touch?). The late Dr. Myles Munroe said, *"The greatest tragedy in life is not death, but a life without a purpose."* Make sure you are making your years count and you have now decided to live life on purpose and make your life count. In doing so, you are showing cancer who's really the boss. For God will always have the last say!

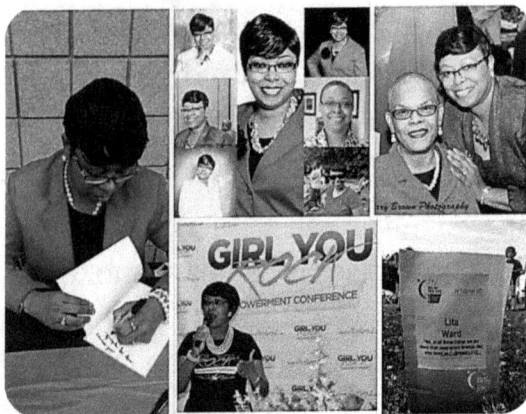

A Word of Encouragement

Currently Diagnosed – *Don't live your life in fear, but live it fearlessly! Remember, you are not a quitter and better days are ahead.*

Conqueror – *Take one day at a time and live in the moment. Grab hold of every opportunity to enjoy life and what it still has to offer.*

Caregiver – *As a caregiver, you have devoted an enormous amount of time and emotional support to your family member or friend. When that person no longer needs you to provide care, it can affect your sense of purpose or self-worth. So, get back to things you may enjoy doing and take care of yourself!*

Conqueror's Notes

"Who shall separate us from the love of Christ? Shall trouble or hardship or persecution or famine or nakedness or danger or sword? ...No, in all these things we are more than conquerors through him who loved us." Romans 8:35, 37 (NIV)

_____

_____

_____

_____

_____

_____

_____

_____

_____

_____

_____

_____

Conqueror's Notes

"Who shall separate us from the love of Christ? Shall trouble or hardship or persecution or famine or nakedness or danger or sword? ...No, in all these things we are more than conquerors through him who loved us." Romans 8:35, 37 (NIV)

Conqueror's Notes

"Who shall separate us from the love of Christ? Shall trouble or hardship or persecution or famine or nakedness or danger or sword? ...No, in all these things we are more than conquerors through him who loved us." Romans 8:35, 37 (NIV)

11

A MUST READ FOR CAREGIVERS

I cannot express how important and essential it is to have a support system while one is going through an illness, a process or anything. Caregivers are even more vital as we pursue our dreams, visions and purpose. Their love, care and service to their loved ones is invaluable and deserve to be noticed. There are also times when the caregiver or support system does not know what to do or how to be supportive. It is no fault of theirs and should be understood that sometimes, they are thrown into these situations without warning and are just afraid of the possible outcome of their family member or friend. As you read the excerpts from some of my family and friends, I am sure you will be able to relate to some of their emotions and see just how blessed I am to have them in my corner, then and now.

My Husband, Mr. Victor J. Ward:

When my wife and I got in the car that Wednesday afternoon to meet with the doctor, we both were overcome with a sense of nervousness as we drove up to the Radiology building's parking lot. Conversation was minimal; I knew she was worried, but I prayed. As we walked into the lobby and was asked to wait for her name to be called for her follow-up appointment, we sat and waited patiently, only anticipating the moment. Then it came; "Lita Ward!" The nurse called out. My wife looked at me and I sensed her fear. "It's going to be alright," I assured her.

We were taken to the back, but into a private room. We knew right then that wasn't a good sign. As soon as we sat down on the room's sofa, I grabbed her hand. Again, waiting to hear what was about to be said. And then the doctor said, "Well, your test is positive; you have Stage 3 cancer in your breast." There were a few seconds of silence, which screamed disbelief! The doctor then tried to assure Lita that she would get through it as she explained the next era of our lives. As her husband and protector, I knew I had to step up to the plate like never before.

On our drive home from the doctor's office, again there was silence in the car, but this time, the quiet was broken with tears streaming down my wife's face. I said to myself, "God give me encouraging words to lift up her spirit; please." We arrived at home and all I could think was this journey was going to be a spiritual battle as we moved forward. Soon as we entered the house, I grabbed her hands and began to pray, knowing that prayer and faith in God was our only hope. After praying, my wife felt more confident that with God's help, she was going to get through this.

Even though we had received this news on our wedding anniversary, we still thought it was an appropriate time to go on vacation in Myrtle Beach, South Carolina. It was a fascinating experience and I noticed my wife's confidence and faith level go through the roof. To see her laughing, joking and having a wonderful time was something I had hoped and longed for. It was an indication that we were ready to take on the fight and get it behind us.

When we returned home, it wasn't long before her chemotherapy treatments began. And it was the most challenging time for both of us; seeing how weak she was at times, not eating, the many sleepless nights at the hospital; reminding her about how beautiful she was even after her hair loss and doing all I could for her during this moment of sickness. It was hard, but I knew I had to stay strong for Lita. Besides God had equipped me for this moment.

I watched my wife grow stronger day by day, as her confidence of recovery increased. Now I look at her and all I can see is the workmanship of God. To look at her now from what she has gone through makes me only glorify God even more. It reminded me that God wants us to play our role in destiny and assured me that all things happen for the good. This experience mended our relationship, bringing us closer to each other and closer to God. We never know what role we must play in life, but the truth of the matter is God prepares us for whatever lies ahead in life. But we cannot be effective unless we believe and trust Him. I thank God for how He used our lives to show His love, His grace and His mercy.

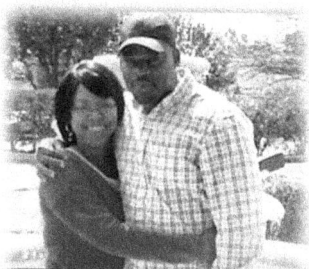

LOVING

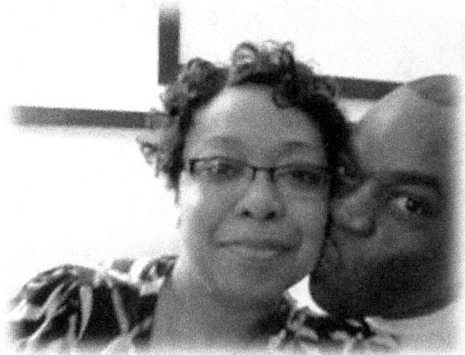

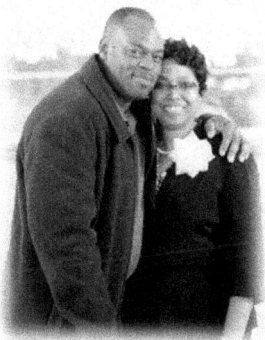

147

From My Daughter, Mrs. Cecelia S. Hoffler:

Worry often tried to creep into my mind as I saw the chemotherapy treatments take their toll on her fragile state. I often found myself leaving my husband's side in the middle of the night, slinking off to the living room to cry and pray in silence. Then one night, he followed me. He told me I didn't have to deal with this alone. We were a team and he was here for me. He held me close and wiped my tears, ensuring me that everything would be okay. That night we prayed and cried together. That night I knew for certain I wasn't dealing with this alone.

Caregivers need care too. As a caregiver for someone who is diagnosed with cancer, never forget to take time to receive care as well. In order to be a strong pillar for your loved one, you must make time to process your own emotions and feelings regarding this life change. Maintaining a brave face in the midst of treatments, fluctuation in health/weight, and mood can prove challenging and downright difficult at times. However, having a support group can make all the difference and aid in your transition to caregiver. I was very fortunate to have a husband who had endured a previous battle with cancer. As a young man, he had been care provider for his grandmother who had conquered cancer. He often shared fond memories of their relationship and how he cared for her till she took her final rest in heaven. The support and counsel he provided my siblings and I during the earlier stages of our mother's treatment were invaluable and brought us all closer together.

Initially devastated at the news of my mother's diagnosis, my mind quickly raced back to every cigarette I purchased and unhealthy activity I personally subjected my body to over the years. And although I had been taught that we ought not to question God's will, the thought still loomed, "Why her?!?!?!" I found myself bitter and angry with God. Why and how could he allow one of the most devout, virtuous women I had ever known to be stricken with cancer? Didn't all her years of service in ministry account for anything? Had she not been faithful enough, endured and suffered enough already? I found myself trying to rationalize and reason with God. "Lord, she's never smoked a day in her life; she actively exercises, eats right and avoids any cancer risk activities."

As I struggled to find words to fully express the weight of the situation, I could only muster up that solitary question, "Why her?" But God is not a god of rationality nor is He a god whose actions perfectly align with our feeble reasoning. For our

149

ways are not His ways and our thoughts are not His thoughts. There was purpose here and as I struggled with understanding the reasoning behind His will for her life, I had to come to the very real conclusion that there was purpose in this pain. An unyielding mind and fervent faith aided in pushing past the palpable pain I often felt when coping with my mother's diagnosis of cancer. With certainty I can proudly say, God has not, cannot and will not fail; only believe.

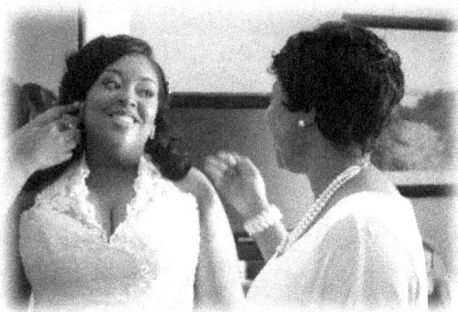

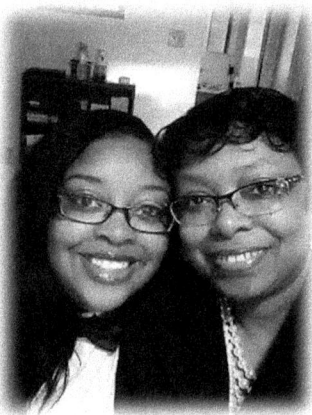

My Son, Mr. Antonio R. Sheppard:

Why do bad things happen to good people? I asked myself that a lot when my mom was diagnosed with breast cancer. I remember hearing those devastating words from dad just like it was yesterday. I suddenly just felt empty inside; I didn't want to lose my mother!

I questioned God as to why and how could this happen to such a loving and amazing woman of God. I know we're not to question God, but at that moment and time, I couldn't help it. I just could not wrap my mind around why her?! Seeing her tired and drained form the chemotherapy treatments made me worry, but I began to pray. I prayed every day; just praying to God that He would heal her. Even though I didn't understand why she had to go through it, that didn't keep me from praying and asking God to please keep my mother here. Seeing that I couldn't help her at all was very painful and I would have given anything to take the cancer away from her. But it wasn't even needed.

Romans 8:28 has stuck with me since that time. "And we know that for those who love God, all things work together for good, for those who are called according to His purpose." So, I ask again, why do bad things happen to good people? Because

God got you regardless. God puts His people in a situation in which He already knows the outcome. You may not understand it, but it's God's plan. In the beginning, I questioned what was God's plan or purpose for allowing this to happen to my mother...but now I know it was *GOD'S PLAN FOR HIS PURPOSE*!

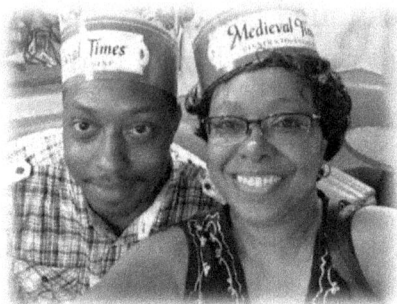

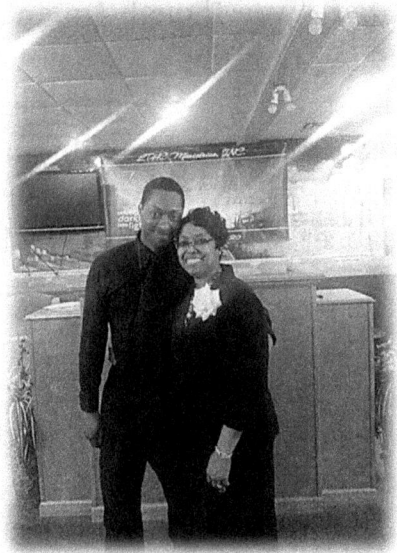

My Son, Mr. Derell Sheppard:

This testament that I'm giving is not one of sorrow, pain, or discouragement. It is one of victory and triumph. Hearing that my mother was diagnosed with breast cancer was one of the most earth-shattering experiences I have ever encountered. This strong woman, so full of life; a woman who raised three children on her own until she remarried. A woman whose faith never wavered in difficult times. I couldn't wrap my mind around her illness; why she had been chosen. Just like my sister, I grew angry with God, questioned His will and logic. Honestly, I thought it was a sick joke at times. I regret feeling that way and allowing my flesh to control my thoughts in that way, but at the end of the day, those were my true feelings.

I've heard a lot of older people say, "Never question God. He knows what He's doing." I've always disliked this statement because how can we find the answer if a question is never proposed? My sister and brother were pillars of strength for me. They never realized how much them being there strengthened me to carry on and be a pillar to my family. I remember when we first heard the news. It was night and my father, Victor Ward, was bringing my brother and I home from work. He broke the news to us and it felt like the temperature dropped 50 degrees below zero. I couldn't believe that cancer had attacked our family; especially the "solitary" of the family. After he had dropped us off, we immediately went to my sister's apartment which was down below ours and we just cried...held each other and cried. The thought of us losing our mother to cancer was more than we could bear individually. We needed to rely on our collective strength. We had to get through it for my mother's sake.

I found myself drinking more from acute depression. Taking several shots to get through the day became routine. Don't get me wrong; I believed God would make everything alright. However, the worry and stress made it easy to rely on alcohol. I didn't know the outcome of this situation and I had no control over it, so I turned to something I thought I could control. I look back on that time as one of the darkest times of my life. Seeing my mother after her chemotherapy treatments and seeing how draining it was on her physically and mentally really hurt my heart. How could I be of help to her? I didn't know anything about being a caregiver in this type of situation. I felt helpless when she would have to go to the hospital and there was nothing I could do. Sometimes I stayed away because I felt like I couldn't do anything to help. I felt powerless seeing my mother go through this battle and I couldn't assist in her struggle. Some days I could see her vitality slip and I feared the worst. I wasn't ready to let go of my mother!

Finding my faith, I prayed, fasted, and believed that God would allow her to stay with me just a little longer. Her struggle would not me in vain and her platform was beginning to manifest in and through her sickness. This chapter of her life became a testament of God's healing power, strength in weakness and faith; not just for others, but for her family as well.

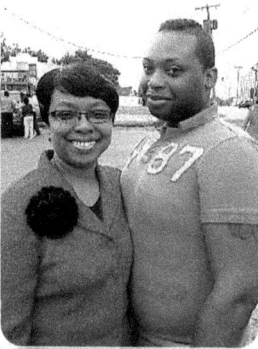

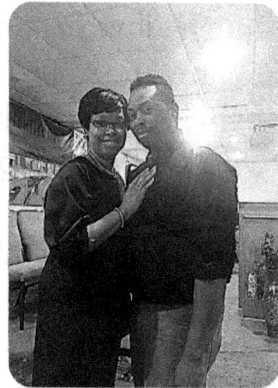

My Friend, Carla R. Cannon:

"The Day Our Lives Changed"

I remember the exact day I received a phone call from Lita sharing that she was diagnosed with breast cancer. I immediately fell on my couch with my mouth wide open in complete shock. Surprisingly Lita seemed to be in much better condition than I was. I remember her voice being calm and she sounded extremely secure in our God that He would see her through.

In that moment, I honestly did not know what to say or do. I remember telling her how much I love her and after our call ended, I dropped to my knees in my living room and wept like a baby. All I was thinking was, *"Why does it seem that bad things often happen to good people?"* I remember calling my Mom crying, saying *"Not my Lita!!!!"* I remember my Mom praying and I felt better. I promise it seemed as if I was in worst shape than Lita was. She sounded super relaxed and unbothered; although I know that wasn't the case, but hey what do you do when the doctor delivers that type of news?

Soon after settling from the news I had to get back to reality and that was with Women of Standard Magazine in which Lita had been the Chief Editor for a few years. I began to ask God,

"What am I to do now?" Lita being the amazing friend she is wanted to continue with the company until it simply became unbearable for her. I remember the moment when she and I were talking on the phone and she said to me, *"I'm afraid that if I leave Women of Standard you will forget all about me."* Those words pierced my soul and of course I immediately responded, *"No way!"*

However, I must admit I wasn't the best friend to Lita throughout this process. Although I prayed for her often and stayed before God on her behalf, she never knew about it. I could have called more, showed up more and simply been there. But I wasn't. Thinking of this brings tears to my eyes but it is my reality.

My best friend was diagnosed with cancer and I was more focused on how I was going to move forward with the magazine that I grew totally consumed with that and raising my daughter while being a "single mom." Truth is, there are no excuses as to why I wasn't there. Sure, I could say I had never had anyone close to me to be sick or diagnosed with any type of disease. Sure, I could say I was in my 20's and I simply lacked wisdom. Or I could say, I didn't know what to do which really was the truth. I was more afraid than anything.

Now that I think back and assess this process, I believe I slowly withdrew from Lita out of fear of losing someone who was so dear to me; which had been the repeated pattern of my life. I am not sure why my mind immediately thought the worst but it did. I thought of my grandmother, Rachel whom I had lost in a car accident when I was twelve years old and I didn't want Lita to be another person I had lost. Sadly, I was more focused on protecting myself rather than being there for her. Unfortunately, this is the reality of our friendship.

However, what I am most grateful for is that Lita extended grace and forgave me. Our friendship has taken its hits with Lita's struggle with effective communication and my struggle with over communicating. *Laughs.* But we have grown through it and vowed to love one another in the midst of it all. I am so grateful for this woman and her strength never cease to amaze me.

Lita P. Ward is an amazing woman whom I am blessed beyond measure to call my friend. We have been blessed to share our journey to Authentic Sisterhood at conferences and there was not a dry eye in the room after we shared our struggles of growing as friends and now as sisters. When I tell you, there is nothing I would not do for her, I mean it; and she knows it.

What Did I Learn?

♦ Experiencing this process with Lita taught me how to be more sensitive to the needs of others. To think less about me and what I had going on and think more about my friend and this life-altering situation at hand.

♦ I also learned that as friends you don't always have to know what to say but it is essential that we be there for our friends. Sure, you can cover one another in prayer, but show up, call them and express the genuine love you have for your friend every chance you get.

♦ Never take anyone you love for granted. Life is short and you never know what may happen. To prevent experiencing any regrets, show love to those you love on a consistent basis.

♦ I learned life is not all about me. Sure, we had to move forward with Women of Standard Magazine and meet deadlines; however, my friend's health and well-being should have meant more than my thoughts of *"What are we going to do now?"*

Lita, I'd like to say thank you for showing the agape love of Jesus and loving me in the midst of my process of learning how to be a better friend.

Because of you I felt first-hand what the love of God really looks like walked out. Thank you for being for me what I once was not to you. Prayerfully by now I have redeemed myself. Ha! Love you girl!

Carla R. Cannon
Catalyst for Change & Speaker to Nations
Periscope|Twitter| IG|FB: @CarlaRCannon
www.CarlaCannon.com

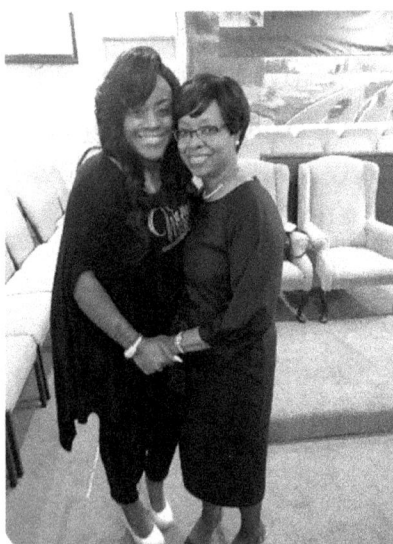

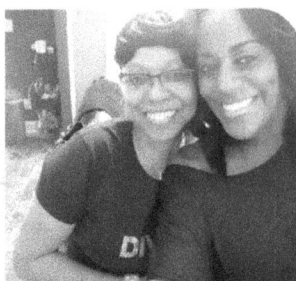

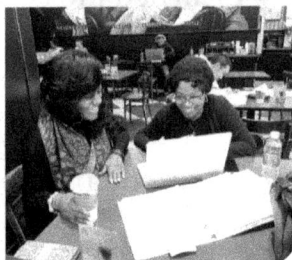

A Word of Encouragement

Currently Diagnosed – *Please be patient with your support system. This is probably new to them and they are just as worried or afraid as you are. Communication is key at this point.*

Conqueror – *When possible, celebrate your caregivers! A card, lunch or just "thank you" for being in your corner during your time of need.*

Caregiver – *Thank you for your love, concern and gift of caring. I commend you for every deed and prayer for your family and friend. If you are currently caring for someone, please visit http://www.cancer.net/coping-with-cancer/caring-loved-one/. It is an excellent website for caregivers.*

12

UNEXPECTED REALITIES

If we believed that everyone is cured or healed from cancer or any disease, we would only be fooling ourselves. More times than we would like to count, loved ones, friends and family succumb to their illnesses. But even though this occurs more than we would like to know, even in death, they are still More Than Conquerors because of their fight until the very end.

Lovingly known by me and too many to name, Sister Icsha (Tammy) Keel was more than a conqueror in her battle with cancer. Icsha and I would not just see and fellowship with each other at our church, but in the waiting room of the Leo Jenkins Cancer Center. She was undergoing treatments for breast cancer as well until it metastasized to her liver. We prayed for one another and encouraged each other to not give up or lose hope. I remember our last conversation, when she told me that cancer had spread to her liver and I was hurt because I was getting better, but she wasn't. Neither did I understand it when she passed away at the age of only 44 years old. I was so wrapped up in grief and guilt that I would not attend her funeral. Instead of consoling her family and our friends, I selfishly chose to console myself and feel guilty.

One thing I did understand though is that Icsha was a beautiful free spirit and she touched many lives with her warm smile and love of life. I learned that I could honor her in living my life to the fullest and reminding myself daily that our time here on earth should be lived to touch and help others. A few years later, her family held a graveside celebration on her birthday and I attended. Not only did I share my feelings, emotions and fears, but I was able to share my love for Icsha and what she meant to me. It was a moment of release and peace, which I will always cherish. Again, she had blessed my life!

Finally, I can say cancer did not take her away from us, but it motivated us to love harder, serve harder and thank God for having experienced His love through my sister and friend, Icsha. Thank you to her loving family for allowing me to remember her as a Conqueror and not a victim. Until we meet again my sister...

MRS. ICSHA TAMMELL BROWN KEEL

"MORE THAN A CONQUEROR"

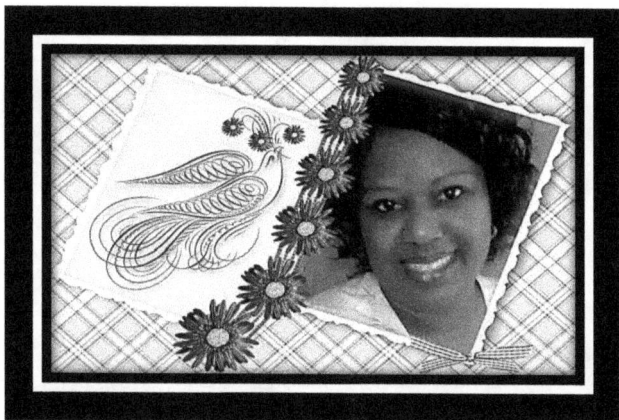

"And if I go and prepare a place for you, I will come again, and receive you unto myself; that where I am, there ye may be also." (John 14:3)

13

CONTINUED JOURNEYS OF MORE CONQUERORS

Brigida Lawrence Morris:

I was just in the prime of my life, my second semester of graduate school and I had met the love of my life. During this time, I noticed a change in a cyst on my left breast that had been previously diagnosed about 10 years ago. I was always encouraged to conduct monthly breast exams and notify my doctor if anything changed. Well around November of 2014, the discomfort became alarming. After a series of testing, on January 6, 2015 I was diagnosed with breast cancer. I can remember sitting in the conference room in the radiologist office thinking this couldn't be happening to me now. I was informed that the cancer was responsive to all types of treatments; however, due to the cyst's size chemotherapy would probably be a part of my treatment plan. So many questions, what next, how would this affect my ability to continue with my graduate program? But never, did I question God as to why this was happening to me.

After my initial diagnosis, I met with the surgical oncologist to find out the specifics about the tumor which included grade and size. I was diagnosed with stage IIB breast cancer. The tumor was about 3 cm in size. My surgical oncologist was very reassuring that things were going to be okay. We further discussed the treatment plan of chemotherapy followed by a lumpectomy. Once meeting with medical oncology, I was informed that my breast cancer was HER2 positive and was provided details regarding the combinations of chemotherapy treatments that I would undergo. I would complete four rounds of chemotherapy to be repeated every three weeks and 12 rounds of Herceptin due to being HER2 positive.

So, one day before Valentine's Day in 2015, I started chemotherapy. Once completing the four rounds of chemotherapy I was prepped for surgery. The surgery was completed with all clear margins with no lymph nodes being affected. Meaning the chemotherapy had killed all the cancer cells. Post-surgery I had a follow with medical oncology. I was excited to be done with chemotherapy so I thought. After speaking with my medical oncologist, she wanted to do three more rounds of chemotherapy due to the initial rounds of chemotherapy not completely shrinking the tumor and because of the cancer being HER2 positive. It was also recommended that I complete genetic testing to further gain insight on ongoing treatment planning.

The last three rounds were tolerated much better than the first four with me only missing one day of work following treatment. I finished the last round of chemotherapy in July 2015 just in time to marry the love of my life in August 2015. Shortly, after I received the test results from the genetic testing and found out that I had the *ATM* gene. This gene is a high-risk gene; however, not as high risk as BRAC1 or BRAC2 genes. I thought all the surgeries were over; however, after speaking with my surgical oncologist we discussed the option of a bilateral mastectomy with reconstructive surgery. I prayed to God for guidance and my husband was supportive of my decision to move forward with plans for surgery. So, in October of 2015 I was scheduled to undergo a bilateral mastectomy with immediate reconstructive surgery. Following the surgery, I had bimonthly visits with the plastic surgeon for breast tissue expander process and in February 2016 I had my final surgery. I will continue to take a hormone therapy medication to reduce reoccurrence for the next five years.

I encourage anyone faced with breast cancer to first have a relationship with God and to surround yourself by those that can intercede on your behalf. You will be faced with so many decisions and have so many fears. It is also important to ensure that you have a dedicated support system that is positive that can be of support to you and give you encouraging words and pray for and with you when you are down. Most of all, I give all thanks to God for trusting in Him and having a personal relationship with Him. It is important to understand that doctors are placed to help guide us through this process from a medical perspective and everything they tell you may not apply to you.

Also, if you know someone who has gone through treatment for breast cancer, talk with them. They can also provide encouraging support. When you are going through treatment, make sure you are taking care of yourself; such as following dietary instructions and most of all avoiding stress. You are dealing with enough with the physical symptoms, psychological symptoms, and day-to-day life. You do not need anything else on top of that. I learned that you just must let go of some things and some people and it is okay to only focus on self during this time.

Looking back, I really wished more information was provided about the physical symptoms other than losing your hair. After taking chemotherapy, there are often lasting side effects which include discoloration of finger and toe nails, change in complexion, and weight gain. And these are only a few I have named. After chemotherapy and my hair began to grow back, my doctor suggested that I refrain from relaxing my hair for about three months. It was hard initially to manage my hair and find appropriate hair care products that worked with my new texture of hair. But as I look into the mirror today, I am so overjoyed to see this beautiful face smiling back at me, healthy and whole.

About Brigida Morris

Brigida L. Morris, MSW, CSAC serves as a Regional Director with a private mental health agency in Greenville, North Carolina. She has over 10 years of experience in assisting children and adults with mental health and substance use needs. In addition, she has worked in settings specific to children and family services.

Mrs. Morris received her Bachelor of Science degree in Family and Community Services from East Carolina University (ECU) and a Masters of Arts degree from Liberty University where she completed the Stress and Trauma Care with Military Application course. Mrs. Morris is a recent graduate from the East Carolina University where she earned a Masters of Social Work degree with a concentration in Substance Use.

Mrs. Morris serves as a team leader on her agency's Critical Incident Stress Management (CISM) team and a training instructor for the local Crisis Intervention Team (CIT). She enjoys spending time with her husband and family; shopping; and vacationing. Mrs. Morris is a member of East Carolina University's Chapter of National Black Social Workers Association and

Alpha Kappa Alpha, Inc. To connect with Brigida, email her at blaw@yahoo.com.

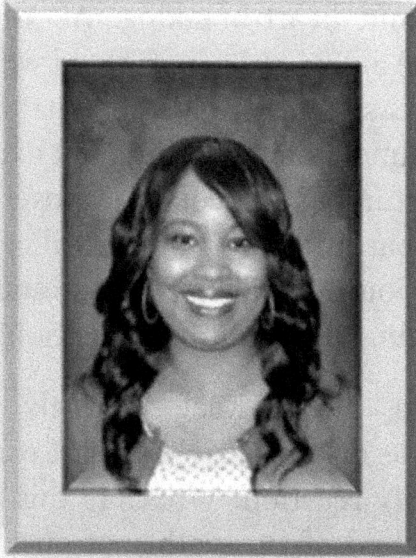

Tyra Abraham:

When you lose someone you love, it can be tough, and it can be painful. When you lose someone you love to cancer, it can be confusing, angering and heart-breaking. All these feelings (and more) are what I experienced when I lost my aunt to breast cancer. This personal encounter is one of misunderstanding, loss, but overall victory. The opportunity to encourage those who have a loved one battling cancer or other illnesses is one I value. The journey will begin at the end: which was the beginning of a beautiful transition!

Icsha Brown-Keel, lovingly known as Tammy, was diagnosed with breast cancer in June of 2007. My reaction: What? Is this a joke? The youngest child of 12, mother of one, and coolest aunt EVER!!? She has what? Personally, I felt that it was caught early and that all would be well. I remember knowing her diagnosis but I don't think the panic came until years later.

I moved back to North Carolina from Virginia in June of 2014 and started working in Greenville. When Auntie's condition begins to worsen, she is admitted to Vidant Medical Center. I visit her on my lunch breaks and after work on most days during her stay. We talk about my upcoming wedding on Nov 15, 2014 and my son (who in her mind can do NO wrong). My insides are screaming, "Lord let her make it to my wedding day! Please God!!" But reality and my nursing judgment do not take back seat to my desire. Because I have been living in another state and have missed so many of her appointments and hospital stays, I feel out of the loop. What is going on? What are the doctors saying? It seemed like overnight her cancer had spread like wildfire. My head is spinning because as a nurse, I'm forcing myself to face reality, but as her niece, I say I need more time. I begin to seek out those who have been by her side daily for more information on her medical status. Like most family, some have a tough time accepting the words of the physicians; other family members can't bring themselves to repeat the prognosis that was given. It's what cancer does. It snatches away hope and replaces it with uncertainty. It makes you angry because "there is nothing that you can do." My burden to bear is the thought of not being more involved. Maybe if I would have visited more often, accompanied her on appointments, talked to her doctors; perhaps this could have gone another way.

July 16, 2014 Wednesday evening: I remember leaving work and going straight to the hospital to see her. She had some balloons and candy in the room from her birthday on Monday.

Whenever Aunt Tammy didn't feel up to talking, I'd just sit at the bedside and chat to her about things that were going on with me. This day was different. I remember feeling like the end was drawing near and I kept forcing myself to grasp that concept. She was having more trouble breathing that day. She was also taken off all monitoring equipment. I didn't realize it then, but deep down I knew I would not see her alive again. I said my goodbye that day when I told her that things here would be taken care of. I said my goodbye that day when we sang the lyrics, "*I guess neither one of us wants to be the first to say goodbye*" (by Gladys Knight). I said my final goodbye when I looked down on her, rubbed her forehead, and uttered how proud I was of her. I remember telling her that she fought bravely so now she needed to take her rest; she deserved it. That moment gives me a great deal of peace. She was scared, understandably, and she was tired.

I left the hospital a little later than usual that evening. It was in the early morning hours of July 17, 2014 when my mom received the call informing her that Auntie was gone. I didn't cry at first. I don't think I cried at all that entire day. We went over to tell my grandmother that her baby girl had passed away. Man that was tough. I must say that my mom did a remarkable job consoling her and

176

keeping her calm. They had just lost a very special person, and together took it like champs (in my book).

Advice to anyone who has a loved one diagnosed with cancer is make the time to be there. There is so much to say and do and if you know the prognosis, make the BEST of the days left. Give them exactly what they want; be supportive as they pass through the stages of death. Second piece of advice I must offer, GET EDUCATED! Educating yourself on your loved one's diagnosis can help you prepare for the days ahead. Consider support groups for family members; they can help tremendously in dealing with feelings you may not know you have. In my experience, I have seen several family members pass away to cancer and other illnesses and their family could not explain what happened. I remember telling my mom, "Take a notebook; write down whatever the doctors say." I encouraged her to write down the date, time, physician's name, and all information that they shared with her. This way, there is a rolling journal, so to speak, that family can refer to if there are any questions. Medical lingo can be so confusing to family and friends: What is that test for? What do the results really mean? Which end of life option should we choose? It can all be overwhelming! Make sure YOU have a support system! YOU will need to find peace in caring for a loved one with cancer and you will need that peace to sustain you after they are gone. My faith in God and prayer has gotten me through one of the toughest losses in my life, my dear Aunt Tammy.

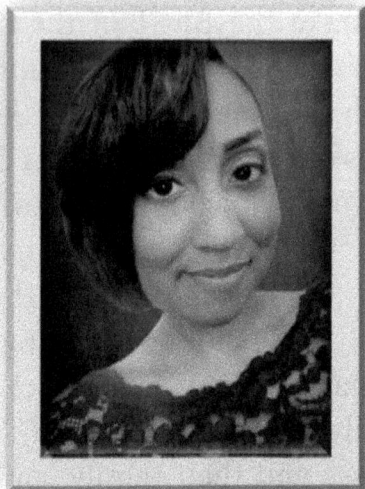

About Tyra Abraham

Tyra Abraham is a nurse with over 10 years of experience in multiple healthcare settings. She describes herself as Kingdom-minded with a heart for God and His people. She is the founder of Duchess League; an organization dedicated to community service and support of its members. The mission of the league is "Ladies with a purpose and passion for helping others, encouraging women, and giving back to communities."

Tyra has lost a lot of family members to cancer, on both sides of her family. She is grateful for the opportunity to share partly of one of those experiences in this book. Tyra resides in Raleigh, NC with her amazing husband, two of their wonderful children, and seven fabulous fish! She enjoys spending time with her family and giving to those in need. To connect with Tyra, visit her organization's website at www.duchessleague.org.

Ivonna Richardson:

In September of 2012, I was heading back to North Carolina on an Amtrak train from Savannah GA. I was returning home from visiting with my dad who was battling life threatening health issues. While sitting on the train I got cold and folded my arms to find warmth. As I was doing this I felt a small pebble size lump under my left arm. The lump was not on the breast but it was right between my arm pit and the left side of my left breast. It wasn't that big but it still alarmed me. I remember thinking to myself, tomorrow will be Monday and I'm calling my doctor first thing in the morning. At the time, I worked at a military health clinic. As soon as I got to work, I reached out to one of the Physicians Assistants. I had her to feel the lump and she said, "I'm sure it's nothing; it's probably just a cyst." I didn't know what to think, but I do know I never ever thought cancer. A few hours later I was able to reach out to my Dr.'s office for a same day appointment. They told me that they wouldn't be able to see me right away, but assured me that the doctor could review this lump at my upcoming annual appointment. But this appointment was 10 days away. I continued to monitor that lump daily to see if it would go away, but it never did. Ten days later I went in to my appointment and the doctor examined my breast. As the previous health professional, he too believed that it was likely a cyst. Besides I was 30 years old, healthy and cancer doesn't run in my family. These were the factors that I kept hearing as professionals assured me that this lump was likely not cancerous. I still wanted tests done, not because I believed that it was cancer because it never crossed my mind. I was very persistent with my doctor because I wanted to find out the cause of this lump. He referred me to the Radiology Department to have an ultrasound and mammogram, which were very uncomfortable. During all of these different procedures, I was still not thinking cancer.

Finally, I was scheduled for the Breast Clinic. I remember sitting waiting for the doctor to come into the exam room. She walked in alongside my nurse and she says, "I'm so sorry Mrs. Richardson, but you have cancer." Tears began to roll down her face, the nurse's face and I'm crying uncontrollably. They both consoled me until I calmed down. Then, the doctor began telling me the protocol for treatment. As I sat there listening, everything was a blur. She discussed chemotherapy, surgeries, staging and radiation. I remember taking the walk from that office to the car and it felt like the loneliest moment in my life. I felt as though I was just given a death sentence. My life and the importance of it began to flash before my eyes in an instance. When I got to the car, the first person I contacted was my mother. We cried on the phone together and she began to encourage me. Then I called my husband, even though at the time we were separated. But he too encouraged me. I stayed in the parking lot of the hospital over an hour just crying and sobbing. I was trying to get myself together to go back to work. I finally contacted my supervisor and told him the news. He encouraged me and told me to go home for the rest of the day. I cried and cried as I drove home. I remember turning from Reilly Road on to Cliffdale Road and I began to feel a peace. My tears began to dry and in that moment, I began to devise a game plan.

The next few months consisted of many appointments. My first surgery was to remove the lump. When the lump was removed, and sent to pathology, it came back as ½ centimeter, Stage I, Triple Negative Breast Cancer. I was told that I would have to do six treatments of chemotherapy, decide if I wanted lumpectomy or mastectomy, and the option for reconstruction. I decided that I would do chemotherapy, following the protocol of

ACT, Adriamycin, Cytoxan, and Taxotere. I chose to have a double mastectomy and reconstruction surgery, which consisted of breast implants. One cool thing about this part was my surgeon gave me the option to choose how large I wanted my new breast to be. I reflected on something that I said in my early twenties. I used to wish that I had bigger breast because I was unsatisfied with my barely B cups and I said I would one day get implants. I chuckled to myself and said, "Lord I didn't mean like this." We must be careful what we wish for because we just might get it, but not in the way we imagined.

My chemotherapy treatment lasted 12 weeks; every other week Wednesday, I would go in for treatments. On Thursdays, a nurse at the clinic that I worked would administer my Neulasta shot, and Fridays I would work half of days. From Friday to Sunday were the days I would be in the worst pain ever. After my first treatment, I decided to visit my beautician to get a short haircut. I thought of this as taking control. I knew the chemotherapy was going to cause hair loss, so I started the process. About 5 days after this, my hair began to fall out. I got into the shower and allowed it all to fall out. Before long every strand of hair that once existed on my body was gone. For many people losing their hair was a hard part of the journey to cope with. I regularly wore hair extensions so this part wasn't easy but it was doable. I struggled with chemotherapy because it was poison entering my body.

I remember having a conversation with God about my fear of this chemotherapy killing me. When I flipped open the Bible, it opened to the book of Mark. As I got to Mark 16:17-18, it read: *"And these signs shall follow them that believe; In my name shall they cast out devils; they shall speak with new tongues; They shall take up serpents; and they shall drink any deadly thing and they shall not die..."* I stood on that Scripture and from that point on, chemotherapy was a breeze because I believed that I had received a divine word from the Lord.

This experience was one of the hardest things that I had to do in my life, requiring me to lean on God more than ever before. Unfortunately, friends and family couldn't comfort me in my darkest moments. At times, I felt alone because I was in another state away from family and friends, and I was going through a separation. I felt as if I wasn't a priority in anyone's life. But, God sent many angels my way to help me get through those times of difficulties. Through this experience, God became a Healer, Friend and Comforter to me. I was prompted by the Holy Spirit to purchase a large red blanket. Anytime I felt hurt, unbearable pain, loneliness, grief or doubt I would swaddle in this blanket. It was symbolic of the blood of Jesus. As I did this, I felt His peace and love comforting me.

Game Plan:

1. I was taught years ago by my Pastor Gary Allen to never claim disease. Never ever say, "My diabetes, my high cholesterol, my cancer." Immediately my mindset shifted. I don't have cancer; I was diagnosed with cancer!

2. I decided that I wouldn't tell everybody about this diagnosis. I only wanted those that would pray and encourage me to know about this fight. Read healing scriptures daily.

3. I began to examine my heart. At the time, I was going through a separation and I had hate, malice and bitterness in my heart. I asked God to help me forgive. As time went on I began to understand that unforgiveness

is like drinking poison and expecting the other person to die. Unforgiveness causes stress and stress is very detrimental to the body. I read the Scripture, *"For our struggle is not against flesh and blood, but against the rulers, against the authorities, against the powers of this dark world and against the spiritual forces of evil in the heavenly realms"* Ephesians 6:12. I would also listen to the song *A Heart that Forgives* by gospel artist Kevin Levar.

4. Let food be thy medicine. I began to make healthier eating choices. I would make green smoothies and stay away from processed foods. I changed my deodorant and other beauty products because of toxic ingredients.

5. Remain Positive. In every tough situation that I encountered, I also found positive things. No matter how negative the situation was I always magnified the positive.

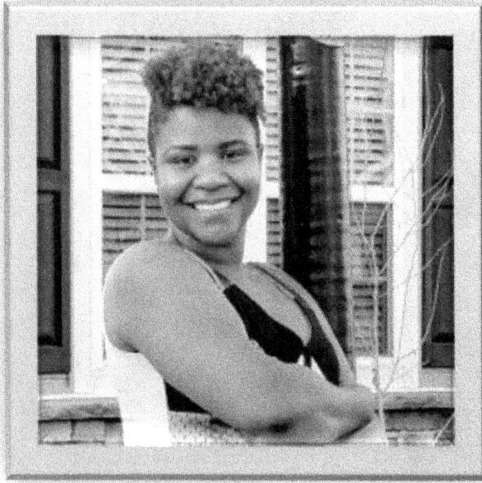

About Ivonna Richardson

Ivonna Richardson was born and raised in Charleston SC; is a military wife, with four beautiful children. She received her undergraduate degree from Ashford University and is currently, pursuing a Master's Degree in Procurement and Acquisitions Management. After receiving the cancer diagnosis in 2012, she decided to leave her position with the Federal Government to pursue her passion for children. Ivonna is now the Owner and Director of Everything Childcare Center in

Fayetteville, NC. To connect with Ivonna, email her at ivonna.richardson@gmail.com.

FREQUENTLY ASKED QUESTIONS

1. Can sex during treatment be harmful to a patient or partner?

According to the American Cancer Society, A few chemotherapy drugs can be present in small amounts in vaginal fluids. You may want to use condoms while you are getting chemotherapy and for about two weeks afterward. Some types of radiation treatment require special precautions for a certain amount of time, too. Talk to your doctor or nurse if you have questions or concerns.

2. What are the symptoms of breast cancer?

- A new lump or mass. However, 80% of lumps are not cancerous.
- A discharge other than breast milk.
- Retraction (inward turning) of the nipple.
- General swelling without a lump.
- Redness in the nipple or breast skin.

3. Are there any foods that increase or decrease your risk of breast cancer?

Yes! The foods and drinks that can lower your risk include: red-orange produce, broccoli, brussels sprouts, cauliflower, beans, lentils, fish rich in omega-3 fatty acids, tofu, and soy milk. The foods and drinks that can raise your risk include: high-fat dairy, sugar, alcohol, and red meat.

4. Does it hurt to have a mammogram?

A mammogram may be slightly uncomfortable, but it shouldn't hurt. In order to get a clear picture, the breast is compressed between two flat plates. It lasts only a few seconds. It is a good idea to schedule a mammogram after your menstrual period when your breasts are less likely to be tender.

5. I've been diagnosed with breast cancer; what's next?

You'll be faced with many decisions you must make and the answers to your questions may not be clear-cut. It's likely you have a little time to make decisions, so don't panic. But don't delay needlessly either; you should be deciding on your course of treatment in the next week or two, after you've gathered the breast cancer support and information you need. If, however, your doctor says your type of cancer requires immediate treatment, your decisions should be made more quickly. So do not waste precious time!

6. What can help me get through this breast cancer treatment process?

- **TAKE TIME FOR YOURSELF.**
This is the time to get plenty of rest, eat right and let other people take care of you.

- **KEEP A JOURNAL OF YOUR CANCER JOURNEY.**
Use your journal to record the specific physiological changes you will go through and your thoughts and fears during the process.

- **EXERCISE.**
You may not feel like running a marathon, but you will feel better mentally as well as physically if you have some physical activity, such as walking or yoga.

- **KEEP THINGS AS NORMAL AS YOU CAN.**
Most people with outside jobs find it's helpful to continue working, although their energy levels might not be high enough for hard chargers to operate at their normal productivity. Many find employers to be very flexible during this time, but make sure you know your rights as an employee.

- **READ TO BE INFORMED AND TO BE INSPIRED.**
  There are many books written by and about breast cancer conquerors such as *More Than A Conqueror*. A few suggestions from me are listed in the appendices section.

7. **Do men ever get breast cancer?**

   According to the American Cancer Society, over 2,200 men are diagnosed with breast cancer in the U.S. each year. Little is known about this rare cancer, but the risk factors seem to be the same as female breast cancer.

8. **How can someone get a second opinion?**

   There are many ways to get a second opinion:

- Ask a primary care provider. He or she may be able to recommend a specialist, such as a surgeon, medical oncologist, or radiation oncologist. Sometimes these doctors work together at cancer centers or programs.

- Call the National Cancer Institute's Cancer Information Service. The number is 800-4-CANCER (800-422-6237). They have information about treatment facilities, including cancer centers and other programs supported by the National Cancer

Institute.

- Seek other options. Patients can get names of doctors from their local medical society, a nearby hospital, a medical school, or local cancer advocacy groups, as well as from other people who have had that type of cancer.

9. How do I break the news to my family?

Informing family and friends can be just as hard as first hearing the news from your doctor. Feelings of concern and worry about upsetting them are normal and expected emotions, which I even experienced. My suggestions are:

- **Be prepared to answer questions.**

They will want to know if you are going to be okay. And they will be just as afraid as you are. So, try to have as much as information you can to help with those questions.

- **Ground and center yourself.**

Before speaking with them, calm your emotions and take time to get your mind and attitude geared in the right direction. If you exhibit a positive attitude, your family should react in a more positive manner.

- **Let someone else speak for you.**

If you cannot bring yourself to talk about it

right now, then ask someone to share the news for you. I asked my husband if he would be the one to tell our children and I asked my sister DeLynn to tell my other sisters, and Mom Glen. I was an emotional basket case and needed their help.

10. Will I ever be *normal* again?

People think that once you are finished with treatments and surgeries, you are fully recovered. But it may take time to recover not just physically, but emotionally as well. If you do not remember anything else, please remember this: **TAKE YOUR TIME!** Your body and mind have been through a lot and the effects of therapy do not necessarily stop when the therapy stops.

Life after breast cancer is, indeed, a different part of life and getting used to whatever it will be takes a while. The journey's easier when women:

- Are honest and open with their loved ones about what they feel.
- Lean on others for the help they need.
- Learn to care for themselves the way they care for others.

AFFIRMATIONS

Affirmations To Overcome Fear

1. I overcome my fear of everything and live life courageously. *(Isaiah 41:10)*

2. I can do all things through Christ who strengthens me! *(Philippians 4:13)*

3. My courage grows as I press on past my fears. *(Deuteronomy 31:6-8)*

4. I now choose love and peace instead of fear. *(2 Timothy 1:7)*

5. Today I use my faith to conquer my fears. *(Galatians 3:9)*

6. I am strengthened and empowered as I challenge my fears. *(Nehemiah 8:10)*

7. My body is healing and improving every day. *(Psalm 30:2)*

8. Everything I need comes to me at the right time. *(Philippians 4:19)*

9. I am strong, fearless and powerful. *(Ephesians 6:10)*

10. Facing my fears empowers me to rise above them. *(Psalm 23:4)*

Affirmations To Overcome Depression

1. I am healthy and whole. *(Isaiah 58:11)*

2. I will try every day to feel good about who I am and what I can be.
   (Romans 12:2)

3. I am grateful for all I am, have, give and receive. *(1 Thessalonians 5:18)*

4. I am grateful for my life, every breath I take, my mind and body. *(Colossians 2:7)*

5. I choose to celebrate and feel gratitude for each day. *(Psalm 9:1)*

6. I inspire others and others inspire me to live a life of wholeness and love.
   (1 Thessalonians 5:11)

7. I have all the guidance, energy, ideas, creativity, power and ability to do all I am meant to do. *(Colossians 2:10)*

8. I am feeling healthy and strong today.
   (Jeremiah 30:17)

9. I am loved, loving and lovable.
   (1 John 4:9-11)

10. My challenges bring me better opportunities.
    (1 Peter 1:6-7)

Affirmations To Overcome Anxiety

1. I easily say no to activities that overburden my schedule. *(Matthew 11:28)*

2. I have the courage to make this a great day. *(John 14:27)*

3. Everything works out for my good! *(Romans 8:28)*

4. My life on earth has meaning and purpose. *(Exodus 9:16)*

5. I trust in God to live a well and fulfilled life. *(Isaiah 26:3)*

6. I am free of anxiety and worry and continue to be so. *(Matthew 6:25-34)*

7. I am free of anything that weighs me down. *(John 8:36)*

8. I will cast all my burdens on the Lord because He cares for me. *(1 Peter 5:7)*

9. The opportunity for peace is always present; therefore, I choose peace. *(John 14:27)*

10. Cancer is something I am temporarily going through. It does not define me or determine my outcome in life. *(2 Corinthians 4:18)*

RECOMMENDED
BOOKS

Ten Books I Recommend

1. *The Holy Bible*

2. *At My Father's Feet* (Lita P. Ward)

3. *A Trailblazer State of Mind: You May Walk Through the Fire But You Shall Not Be Burned* (Carla R. Cannon)

4. *Cancer, Cancelled For The Glory of God* (Angel B. Staton)

5. *I Flunked My Mammogram: what every woman needs to know about breast cancer* (Ernie Bodai, M.D. and Richard Zmuda)

6. *No Way To Lose* (Bishop Rosie S. O'Neal)

7. *The Cancer Book, Chicken Soup for the Soul* (Jack Canfield, Mark Hansen & David Tabatsky)

8. *The Confident Woman Devotional* (Joyce Meyer)

9. *What Happens To Good People When Bad Things Happen* (Robert A. Schuller)

10. *Your Best Is Yet To Come* (Parris Solomon)

APPENDICES

Appendix I:

Glossary

of

Terms

Appendix I:

Glossary of Terms

These are some words/terms you may hear your healthcare team use.

A

Adjuvant therapy: Treatment used in addition to main treatment. Usually refers to hormone therapy, chemo, radiation, or immunotherapy given after surgery to increase the chances of curing the disease or keeping it in check.

Alopecia: Hair loss, which can be all over the body. It is often caused by chemo, but hair usually grows back.

Anti-emetic: A medicine to prevent or control nausea and vomiting.

Antibiotics: Drugs used to treat infection.

Areola: The darkened area surrounding the nipple.

Arimidex: A drug used to treat certain types of breast cancer in postmenopausal women. By lowering the amount of estrogen made by the body, this may stop the growth of cancer cells that need estrogen.

Axilla: The underarm.

Axillary: Pertaining to the underarm.

Axillary dissection: Surgery to remove lymph nodes under the arm.

B

Benign: Not cancerous; does not spread to other parts of the body

Biopsy: The removal of a piece of tissue taken from the body to examine it more closely for cancer cells.

Bone density: A measurement of the amount of calcium and other minerals in a segment of bone, a higher mineral content indicating a higher bone density and strength, used to detect osteoporosis or monitor its treatment.

BRCA1: A gene that normally acts to restrain the growth of cells in the breast but which, when mutated, predisposes to breast cancer. The gene's full name is breast cancer 1, early onset.

BRCA2: A gene that increase risks for breast cancer; proteins from this gene and the BRCA1 are essential for repairing damaged DNA.

Breast Construction: A surgical procedure that restores shape to your breast after mastectomy — surgery that removes your breast tissue to treat or prevent breast cancer.

C

Cancer: A term for diseases in which abnormal cells divide without control and can invade nearby tissues. Cancer cells can also spread to other parts of the body through the blood and lymph systems.

Carcinogen: Any substance that is known to cause cancer.

Cell: The structural and functional unit of all living organisms, and is sometimes called the "building block of life."

Chemotherapy: A drug treatment that uses powerful chemicals to kill fast-growing cells in the body. Chemotherapy is most often used to treat cancer, since cancer cells grow and multiply much more quickly than most cells in the body.

Clinical Trials: Research studies that involve patients, which are carefully designed to find better ways to prevent, detect, diagnose and treat cancer.

Combination chemotherapy: The use of more than one chemo drug to treat cancer.

Corticosteroid: Any steroid hormone used as hormone replacement, to suppress the immune system, and to treat some side effects of cancer and its treatment.

D

Dexamethasone: A drug used to reduce inflammation and lower the body's immune response or treat many other diseases and conditions related to cancer. Dexamethasone is a type of corticosteroid.

DNA (deoxyribonucleic acid): The hereditary material in humans; a large molecule that carries the genetic information that cells need to replicate and produce proteins.

Diagnosis: The process of identifying a disease, condition, or injury from its signs and symptoms.

A health history, physical exam, and tests, such as blood tests, imaging tests, and biopsies, may be used to help make a diagnosis.

Duct: A tube in the body that fluids pass through.

Ductal carcinoma in situ: Abnormal cells inside a duct in the breast, considered being the earliest form of breast cancer. It is non-invasive, meaning it hasn't spread outside of duct to invade other parts of the breast.

E

Estrogen: A hormone that occurs naturally in women; also promotes tumor growth.

External Radiation: A method of radiation therapy for delivering a beam or several beams of high-energy x-rays to a patient's tumor.

F

Fatigue: The feeling of being tired physically, mentally and emotionally. Cancer-related fatigue persists over time and interferes with usual activities.

Fluorouracil (5-FU): It is a medication, which is used in the treatment of cancer. Trade name is Adrucil among others.

G

Gene: The basic physical and functional unit of heredity.

Gland: An organ that makes one or more substances, affecting tissues or organs. Others producing hormones or participating in blood production.

Grade: Description of a tumor based on how abnormal the tumor cells and the tumor tissue look under a microscope. It is an indicator of how quickly a tumor is likely to grow and spread.

Grading: A system for classifying cancer cells in terms of how abnormal they appear when examined under a microscope. It provides information about the growth rate of the tumor and its tendency to spread and plays a role in treatment decisions.

H

HER-2/neu: A protein involved in normal cell growth. It is found on some types of cancer cells, including breast and ovarian. Cancer cells removed from the body may be tested for the presence of HER2/neu to help decide the best type of treatment.

Hormonal therapy: Treatment that adds, blocks, or removes hormones; specifically, to slow or stop the growth of cancer.

Hormones: They are natural substances released by an organ that can influence the functions of other organs in the body and the growth of some types of cancer.

I

Immune system: A complex network of cells, tissues, organs, and the substances they make that helps the body fight infections and other diseases. The immune system includes white blood cells and organs and tissues of the lymph system.

Immunotherapy: A type of biological therapy that uses substances to stimulate or suppress the immune system to help the body fight cancer.

Inflammatory: Having to do with inflammation (redness, swelling, pain, and a feeling of heat that helps protect tissues affected by disease).

Inflammatory breast cancer: A type of breast cancer in which the breast looks red and swollen and feels warm. The skin of the breast may also show the pitted appearance like the skin of an orange. The redness and warmth occur because the cancer cells block the lymph vessels in the skin.

In situ: In its original place. For example, in carcinoma in situ, abnormal cells are found only in the place where they first formed and have not spread.

Intravenous: A way of giving a drug or other substance through a needle or tube inserted into a vein. Also called IV.

Invasive breast cancer: Cancer that has spread from where it began in the breast to surrounding normal tissue. Also called infiltrating breast cancer.

L

Lobular carcinoma in situ: A condition in which abnormal cells are found in the lobules of the breast. This condition seldom becomes invasive cancer. However, having lobular carcinoma in situ in one breast increases the risk of developing breast cancer in either breast. Also called LCIS.

Lumpectomy: An operation to remove the cancer and some normal tissue around it, but not the breast itself. Some lymph nodes under the arm may be removed for biopsy.

Lymph nodes: Lymph nodes filter substances that travel through the lymphatic fluid, and they contain lymphocytes (white blood cells) that help the body fight infection and disease. Clusters of lymph nodes are found in the neck, underarm, chest, abdomen, and groin. Also called lymph glands.

Lymphedema: A condition in which extra lymph fluid builds up in tissues and causes swelling. It may occur in an arm or leg if lymph vessels are blocked, damaged, or removed by surgery, or blocked by cancer cells.

M

Magnetic resonance imaging: A procedure in which radio waves and a powerful magnet linked to a computer are used to create detailed pictures of areas inside the body. These pictures can show the difference between normal and diseased tissue. Also called an MRI.

Malignant: Cancerous. Malignant cells can invade and destroy nearby tissue and spread to other parts of the body.

Mammogram: An x-ray of the breast.

Mammography: The use of x-ray, film or a computer to create a picture of the breast.

Mastectomy: Surgery to remove part or the entire breast.

Menopausal hormonal therapy: Treatment with the hormones estrogen and progesterone or with estrogen alone to help relieve symptoms of menopause. Symptoms may include hot flashes, night sweats, vaginal dryness, sleep problems, mood swings, and thinning of the bones. Menopausal hormone therapy is given to replace the natural hormones that are no longer made by the body. It is given to women who have gone through menopause or who have early menopause caused by cancer treatment or by having their ovaries removed by surgery. Also called MHT.

Menopause: The time of life when a woman's ovaries stop producing hormones and menstrual periods stop. Natural menopause usually occurs around age 50.

Metastasize: To spread from one part of the body to another. When cancer cells metastasize, and form secondary tumors, the cells in the metastatic tumor are like those in the original (primary) tumor.

O

Oncologist: A doctor who has special training in diagnosing and treating cancer.

Oncology: A branch of medicine that specializes in the diagnosis and treatment of cancer. It includes medical oncology (the use of chemotherapy, hormone therapy, and other drugs to treat cancer), radiation oncology (the use of radiation therapy to treat cancer), and surgical oncology (the use of surgery and other procedures to treat cancer).

P

Pathologist: A doctor who has special training in identifying diseases by studying cells and tissues under a microscope.

Pathology report: The description of cells and tissues made by a pathologist based on microscopic evidence, and sometimes used to make a diagnosis of a disease.

Peripheral neuropathy: Damage to the nervous system that usually begins in the hands and/or feet with symptoms of tingling, numbness, burning, and/or weakness. Some chemo drugs can cause it.

Platelets: Special blood cells that plug up damaged blood vessel and help blood clot to stop bleeding.

Precancerous: A term used to describe a condition that may or is likely to become cancer.

Progesterone: A female hormone made by the body that plays a role in the menstrual cycle and pregnancy.

Prognosis: The likely outcome or course of a disease; the chance of recovery or recurrence.

R

Radiation therapy: The use of high-energy radiation from x-rays, gamma rays, and other sources to kill cancer cells and shrink tumors.

Radiologist: A doctor who has special training in creating and interpreting pictures of areas inside the body. The pictures are made with x-rays, sound waves, or other types of energy.

Radiology: The use of radiation (such as x-rays) or other imaging technologies (such as ultrasound and magnetic resonance imaging) to diagnose or treat disease.

Recurrence: Cancer that has recurred (come back), usually after a period of time during which the cancer could not be detected. The cancer may come back to the same place as the original (primary) tumor or to another place in the body.

Remission: Disappearance of signs and symptoms of cancer, meaning that tests, physical exams, and scans show that all signs of cancer are gone.

Risk factor: Something that increases the chance of developing a disease. Some examples of risk factors for cancer are age, a family history of certain cancers, use of tobacco products, being exposed to radiation or certain chemicals, infection with certain viruses or bacteria, and certain genetic changes.

S

Screening: Checking for disease when there are no symptoms. Since screening may find diseases at an early stage, there may be a better chance of curing the disease. Examples of cancer screening tests are the mammogram (breast), colonoscopy (colon), and the Pap test and HPV test (cervix).

Side effects: A problem that occurs when treatment affects healthy tissues or organs. Some common side effects of cancer treatment are fatigue, pain, nausea, vomiting, decreased blood cell counts, hair loss, and mouth sores.

Staging: Performing exams and tests to learn the extent of the cancer within the body, especially whether the disease has spread from the original site to other parts of the body.

Stomatitis: Sores on the lining of the mouth

T

Topical: To put right on the skin

Tumor marker: A substance found in tissue, blood, or other body fluids that may be a sign of cancer. A tumor marker may help to diagnose cancer, plan treatment, or find out how well treatment is working or if cancer has come back.

U

Ultrasound: A procedure that uses high-energy sound waves to look at tissues and organs inside the body. The sound waves make echoes that form pictures of the tissues and organs on a computer screen (sonogram). Ultrasound may be used to help diagnose diseases, such as cancer.

W

White blood cells: The blood cells that fight infection.

Conqueror's Notes

"Terms I Need to Ask My Doctor or Nurse About..."

_____

_____

_____

_____

_____

_____

_____

_____

_____

_____

_____

_____

Conqueror's Notes

"Terms I Need to Ask My Doctor or Nurse About..."

_____

_____

_____

_____

_____

_____

_____

_____

_____

_____

_____

_____

Conqueror's Notes

"Terms I Need to Ask My Doctor or Nurse About..."

_____

_____

_____

_____

_____

_____

_____

_____

_____

_____

_____

_____

_____

Appendix II:

References

Appendix II:

References

The following references were used to compile the information presented and are great resources to assist you or your loved one on their journey to wellness.

American Cancer Society. (2006). Nutrition for the Person with Cancer during Treatment [Brochure]. Greenville, NC. www.cancer.org

American Cancer Society. (2009). Understanding Chemotherapy [Brochure]. Greenville, NC. www.cancer.org

Bauer, A. (2014, June 26). The Power of Writing. Retrieved November 07, 2016, from http://www.cancer.net/blog

Bodai, E., & Zmuda, R. A. (2005). "I flunked my mammogram!": What every woman needs to know about breast cancer (2nd ed.). Severna Park, MD: B2Z Pub.

Breastcancer.org - Breast Cancer Information and
Awareness. (n.d.). Retrieved July/August,
2016, from http://www.breastcancer.org/

Caring for a Loved One. (2016, November 10).
Retrieved March 01, 2017, from
http://www.cancer.net/coping-with-
cancer/caring-loved-one/.

National Institutes of Health (NIH) | Turning
Discovery Into Health. (n.d.). Retrieved
November 01, 2016, from
https://www.nih.gov/.

Phone, B. (n.d.). Living Beyond Breast Cancer.
Retrieved November 06, 2016, from
http://www.lbbc.org/.

Susan G. Komen | Susan G. Komen®. (n.d.).
Retrieved September 22, 2016, from
http://ww5.komen.org/.

The Holy Bible: Authorized King James Version.
(2003). Nashville, TN: Thomas Nelson.

Conqueror's Personal Journal

This is your place and space to record your thoughts, feelings or whatever your heart desires. One day you will look back and see just how far you have come on your journey to wellness.

I can shake
off everything
as I write,
my sorrows
disappear,
my courage
is reborn.

— Anne Frank

PERSONAL JOURNAL

PERSONAL JOURNAL

PERSONAL JOURNAL

PERSONAL JOURNAL

PERSONAL JOURNAL

_____

_____

_____

_____

_____

_____

_____

_____

_____

_____

_____

_____

_____

_____

PERSONAL JOURNAL

PERSONAL JOURNAL

PERSONAL JOURNAL

PERSONAL JOURNAL

PERSONAL JOURNAL

_____

_____

_____

_____

_____

_____

_____

_____

_____

_____

_____

_____

_____

_____

PERSONAL JOURNAL

_____

_____

_____

_____

_____

_____

_____

_____

_____

_____

_____

_____

_____

PERSONAL JOURNAL

Meet the Author

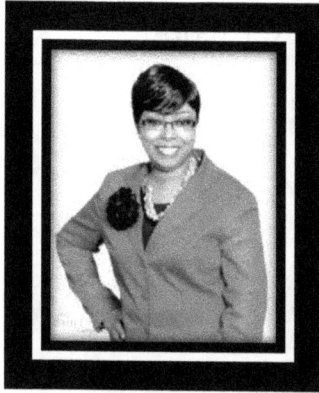

Lita P. Ward is an ordained evangelist, author of three books, and COO of LPW Editing & Consulting Services, which provides professional editing, formatting and proofreading for authors, students, businesses and job seekers. There is no job too small or large for her company. Their mantra is *Inspired by Vision; Driven by Purpose.* LPW Editing & Consulting Services ensures that once a client's project leaves their hands, the product is polished and professional.

She is the Director of Women of Standard Network and Chief Editor of Cannon Publishing. Also, Lita is the Location Director and Adjunct Instructor at the University of Mount Olive in Washington, North Carolina, where she oversees the day-to-day operations and teaches religion and student success to the non-traditional population her institution caters to. She resides in Greenville, NC with her husband, Victor J. Ward. Connect with Lita at www.litaward.org.

www.ingramcontent.com/pod-product-compliance
Lightning Source LLC
Chambersburg PA
CBHW052124270326
41930CB00012B/2750